ART, FAITH AND MEDICINE IN TINTORETTO'S VENICE

edited by

Gabriele Matino

Cynthia Klestinec

Marsilio

SAVE VENICE

ART, FAITH AND MEDICINE IN TINTORETTO'S VENICE

Scuola Grande di San Marco, Venice
September 6, 2018 – January 6, 2019

Exhibition organized and produced by
SAVE VENICE

Azienda Ulss3 Serenissima
REGIONE DEL VENETO
ULSS3 SERENISSIMA

Polo Culturale e Museale
Scuola Grande di San Marco
SCUOLA GRANDE DI SAN MARCO 580 1438 · 2018

With the scientific collaboration of
Archivio di Stato di Venezia

With the patronage of
Curia Patriarcale di Venezia

With additional support from
The Thompson Family Foundation, Inc.
The Gladys Krieble Delmas Foundation
through Save Venice Inc.

Catalogue published thanks to
Save Venice Inc.
with a contribution from
The Gladys Krieble Delmas Foundation

Installation Project
Guido Jaccarino
Federico Marcato

Installation
Uni.S.Ve. srl
Gino Feltrin
Gruppo Fallani s.r.l.

Condition Report
Laura Martini

Lighting
Luca Marchiò for SIRAM S.p.A.

Videos during Exhibition
Department of Exhibition Program
National Gallery of Art,
Washington, DC
videoinmov

Art Handling
Uni.S.Ve. srl

Insurance
Generali Italia S.p.A.
Agenzia Generale, Carpenedo

Graphic Project
Giorgio Tommasi
Federico Marcato

Conservators
Giulia Barbero
Barbara Biciocchi
Conservation by Design LTD
Jarmila Kodrič
Laura Martini
Valentina Piovan
Paola Santin Conservazione e restauro

Save Venice Inc. thanks all those who made the exhibition possible, especially the lending institutions, the museums, and their directors:

Ministero dei beni e delle attività culturali e del turismo
Direzione generale Musei
Director General
Antonio Lampis
Director Servizio I - "Collezioni Museali"
Antonio Tarasco
Declaration of Relevant Cultural Interest
Silvia Trisciuzzi

Soprintendenza Speciale per il Patrimonio Storico, Artistico ed Etnoantropologico per il Polo Museale della Città di Venezia e dei Comuni della Gronda Lagunare
Director
Emanuela Carpani

Archivio di Stato di Venezia
Director
Giovanna Giubbini

Biblioteca Nazionale Marciana
Director
Maurizio Messina

Curia Patriarcale di Venezia
Patriarchal Delegate for Cultural Heritage
Gianmatteo Caputo

Fondazione Giorgio Cini Onlus
Biblioteca Manica Lunga
Coordinator
Simone Guerriero

Fondazione Musei Civici di Venezia
Director
Gabriella Belli

Galerie Arnoldi-Livie, Monaco
Director
Cornelia Muessing

Gallerie dell'Accademia di Venezia
Director
Paola Marini

Istituto Ortopedico Rizzoli di Bologna
Director General
Mario Cavalli
Scientific Director
Maria Paola Landini

Save Venice Inc. and the curators also thank:
Antea Boscarato
Patricia Fortini Brown
Lorenzo Buonanno
Tracy Cooper
Tiarna Doherty
Robert Echols
Cristina Fusetti
Frederick Ilchman
Sarah Blake McHam
Theodore Rabb
Adam Tessier
Irina Tolstoy

Actv

Media sponsor
AracneTV
Jerusalem
RIVISTA DI ARCHITETTURE PER LO SPIRITO

THERE IS A significant manner in which this exhibition is in keeping with our health service's fundamental mission of care: it in fact makes clear the principle of integration of different human events that are usually considered decidedly distinct but above all are seen as distant from one another. Faith, art, and medicine have, however, a single basis in the quest for salvation, through redemption, beauty, and healing.

We often feel a strong need to find someone and something to remind us that care of the body of others is service (*therapeia*); and if it is service it is obedience, namely the exercise of listening (*ob-audire*) to the sick person. Thus the beauty that we look for in art is the representation of a balance of anatomical forms but also a quest for the self, a going beyond to find truer ethical beauty. But it is in faith that we are most authentically listening, because we are seeking the divine; in the relationship with the *logos* our words sound genuine when they declare the limits of a humanity that asks for life.

We have the privilege of preserving here in Venice at a single site — the Scuola Grande di San Marco — signs of all three of these realities. They are the most profound that humanity has produced over the thousands of years of its history and ones that, if shown in all their authenticity, offer the right understanding of the person in its integrity: need for transcendence, expectation of health, fear of illness, desire for self-realization, selflessness, openness to charity (*charitas*), and more. At the same time, these signs demonstrate a value that is truly rare in the panorama of museum culture, and not just in Italy; signs that time has laid down in this place, in the Scuola Grande di San Marco and its building, the works of art housed in it, its collections of the history of medicine.

All this goes hand in hand, in an enriching and uncommon manner, with the living medical practice that the hospital of the Venetians has been offering on a daily basis for centuries, originally at a location close to the Scuola, subsequently inside it and today in harmony with it. Thus the paradigm of life is complete and that service is also proposed as a moral virtue of the community.

This singular situation finds expression at the highest level in the exhibition that we are hosting in the Sala Capitolare of the Scuola. For this we must thank Save Venice Inc., which had the idea of staging this event on our premises, bearing witness once again to the regard and affection that it holds for our institution and its historical and artistic works. We must also express our gratitude to the bodies and scholars that have organized the exhibition, effectively connecting for the first time paintings, books, documents, and antique objects that all have their origin and inspiration in our Scuola. We are grateful, finally, to the Italian and foreign institutions that have agreed to our requests for the loan of works: it is an important mark of the credibility that the Museum and Cultural Center of the Scuola Grande di San Marco has acquired in a short space of time among its many friends in this city and the world, following its establishment just five years ago.

We offer, to residents of the city and to every visitor, a cultural insight into the person that is not abstract, not forgetful of the past, and not fearful of a future without fathers.

Giuseppe Dal Ben
Director General
Azienda ULSS 3 Serenissima

Mario Po'
Director
Polo Culturale e Museale
Scuola Grande di San Marco, Venice

PERHAPS MORE THAN any Italian painter of the sixteenth century, and certainly more than any Venetian one, Jacopo Tintoretto (c. 1519–94) perfected the depiction of the muscular human body in action. Even when engaged in miraculous activities, the figures that populate Tintoretto's enormous canvases seem to breathe air and move through space in a way that we find completely convincing. Although an artist rather than a physician or surgeon, Tintoretto had a deep familiarity with human anatomy and the movements of the body. Yet in his day Tintoretto was not alone in his fascination with the natural world. Many Venetians benefitted from the growing medical knowledge of the sixteenth century and its dissemination through charitable and educational institutions. Their lives reconciled religious faith and medical knowledge. Venice was simultaneously a center of scientific discovery and Christian piety, and this combination was woven into the social fabric of the city and its mainland territories.

Save Venice is proud to organize and serve as the sole sponsor of *Art, Faith and Medicine in Tintoretto's Venice*, an initiative in honor of the 500th anniversary of the birth of Jacopo Tintoretto. This exhibition and publication advance our organization's mission of educating the public about diverse aspects of Venice's priceless cultural heritage. Held at the Scuola Grande di San Marco, this innovative exhibition of medical history had its starting point in the Scuola's multiple historical identities as a religious institution, a site of care for the ill, and a monument of Renaissance art and architecture particularly associated with Tintoretto. One of six major lay confraternities in Venice, the Scuola provided spiritual and physical care to the sick and dying as a centerpiece of its charitable mission. Today, the building serves as the entrance to the city's modern hospital and houses an important library of historical medical books and manuscripts. The structure is one of the most magnificent in the city, with a sumptuous façade of marble and Istrian stone — restored by Save Venice in 2000–2005 — and meeting rooms with spectacular carved and gilded ceilings. The walls of its Chapter Hall were originally decorated with a cycle of paintings depicting miracles of Saint Mark. The first canvases of this landmark ensemble were created by Jacopo Tintoretto — among them his breakthrough work, the *Miracle of the Slave* (1548) — and the cycle was completed by Jacopo's son Domenico. Four of Domenico's paintings, conserved by Save Venice between 2004 and 2014, remain on site, along with the altarpiece by Jacopo Palma il Giovane, another Save Venice restoration. How fitting, then, that as part of the celebration of the birth of Jacopo Tintoretto, that great painter of the dynamic human body, the Scuola should be the site of this exhibition that explores and illuminates the many interconnections among art, religious faith, and medical science in sixteenth-century Venice.

The exhibition includes a conservation component: Save Venice provided funding for treatment of eighteen important manuscripts and books so that they could be displayed here and also preserved for future generations. Among these conserved treasures are the oldest surviving visual document relating to the Scuola, a fourteenth-century double miniature attributed to the artist Paolo Veneziano, from the confraternity's original rule book (*mariegola*), and a copy of the famous anatomical treatise by Vesalius owned by Tommaso Rangone, who figures prominently in the history of this institution and within this exhibition as a notable physician, officer of the Scuola, and an important patron of Tintoretto.

Save Venice is deeply grateful to the numerous institutions in Venice and elsewhere that lent works and provided support, above all the Scuola Grande di San Marco and Ospedale di Venezia. Special thanks are due to Dottore Giuseppe Dal Ben, director general, Azienda Ulss 3 Serenissima, and Dottore Mario Po', director, Polo Culturale e Museale Scuola Grande di San Marco. The exhibition was made possible in part by a generous grant to Save Venice from The Thompson Family Foundation, while the Gladys Krieble Delmas Foundation funded this catalogue and additional exhibition expenses.

The exhibition was curated by scholars Gabriele Matino and Cynthia Klestinec, co-editors of the catalogue and specialists in Venetian art history and Renaissance anatomy and dissection respectively. They were joined by Melissa Conn, Director of the Venice office of Save Venice, who coordinated all aspects of the budget, finances, and institutional relations. Guidance and assistance were provided by the distinguished members of the Committee of Honor and the scholarly Advisory Committee. A number of members of the board of directors of Save Venice, among them Patricia Fortini Brown, Tracy Cooper, Sarah Blake McHam, and Theodore Rabb, particularly championed this project and helped with the catalogue. The initial idea for the exhibition was proposed by Save Venice Chairman Frederick Ilchman, D. Dodge Thompson, Head of Exhibitions at the National Gallery of Art, Washington, and co-curator Gabriele Matino.

Save Venice invites you to explore, through this exhibition and publication, yet another aspect of the extraordinary history of our beloved city.

Irina Tolstoy
Chair, Educational Resources Committee
Save Venice Inc.

Translations
Huw Evans

Graphic Design and Layout
Tomomot, Venezia

Editing
Enrico Cioni

Cover
Domenico Tintoretto, *Dream of Saint Mark*,
c. 1587–90. Oil on canvas, Venice,
Gallerie dell'Accademia. Detail.

First edition August 2018
ISBN 978-88-317-2947-5

www.marsilioeditori.it

Available through ARTBOOK | D.A.P.
75 Broad Street, Suite 630 New York, NY 10004
www.artbook.com

CONTENTS

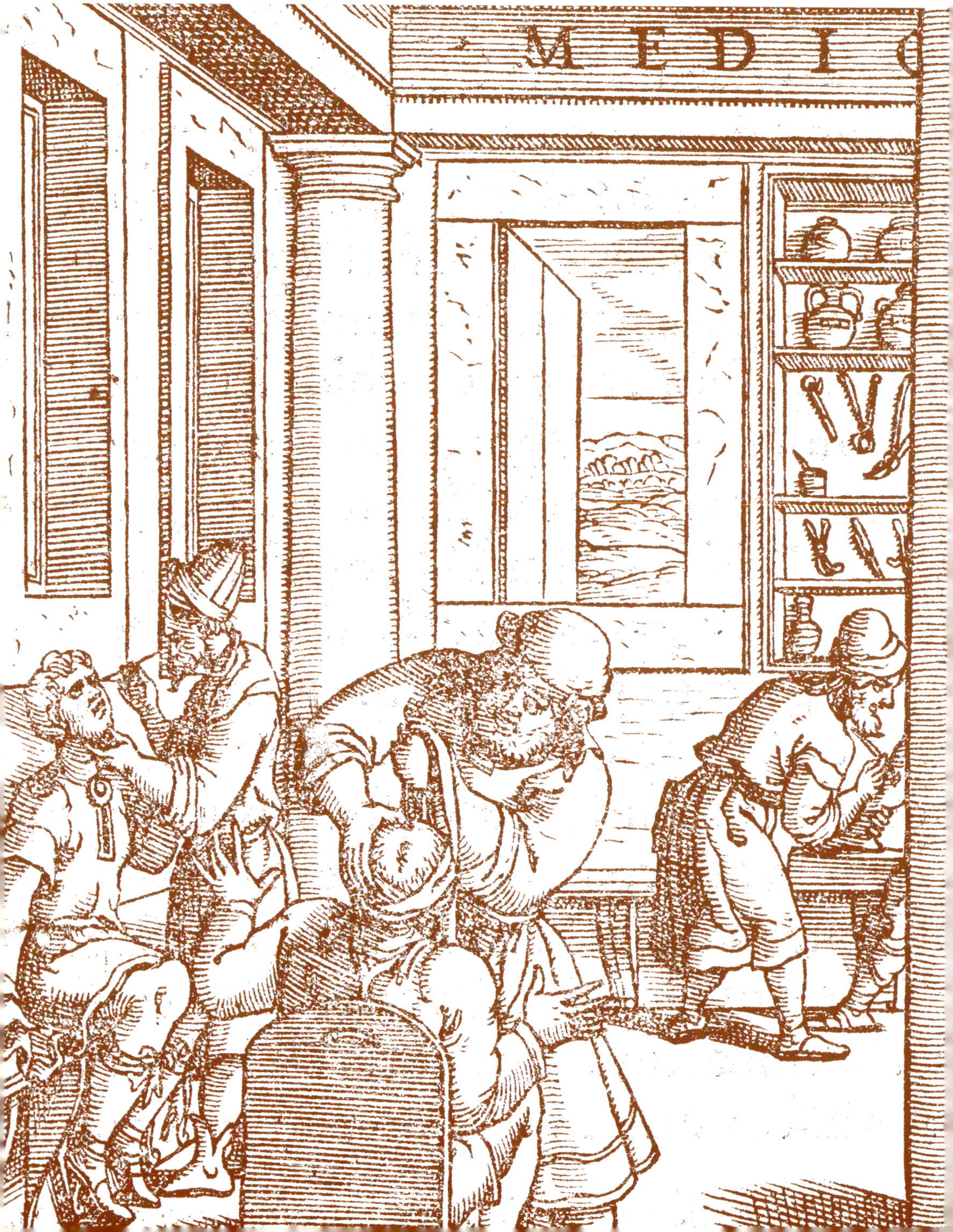
MEDIC

ART, FAITH AND MEDICINE
IN TINTORETTO'S VENICE

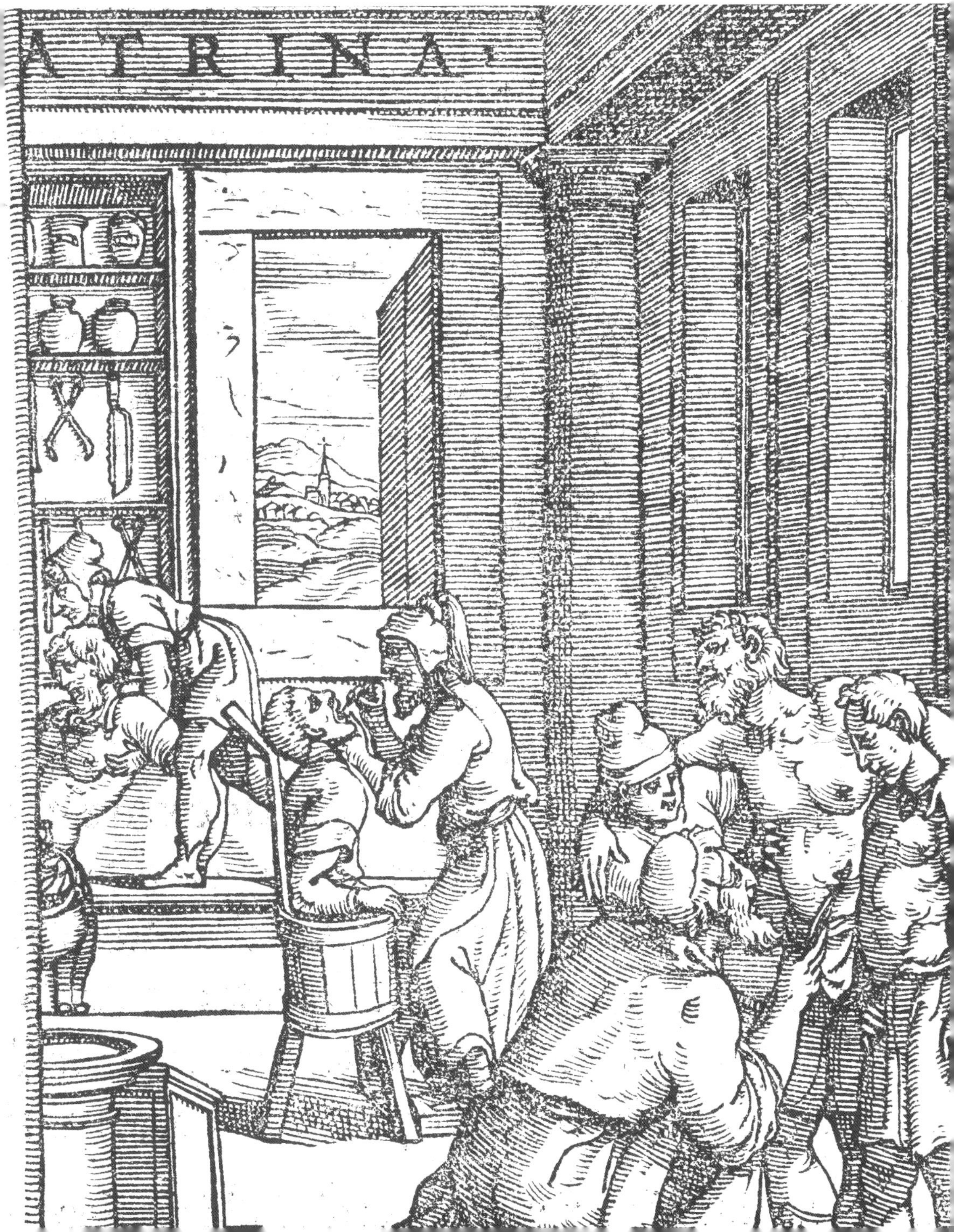

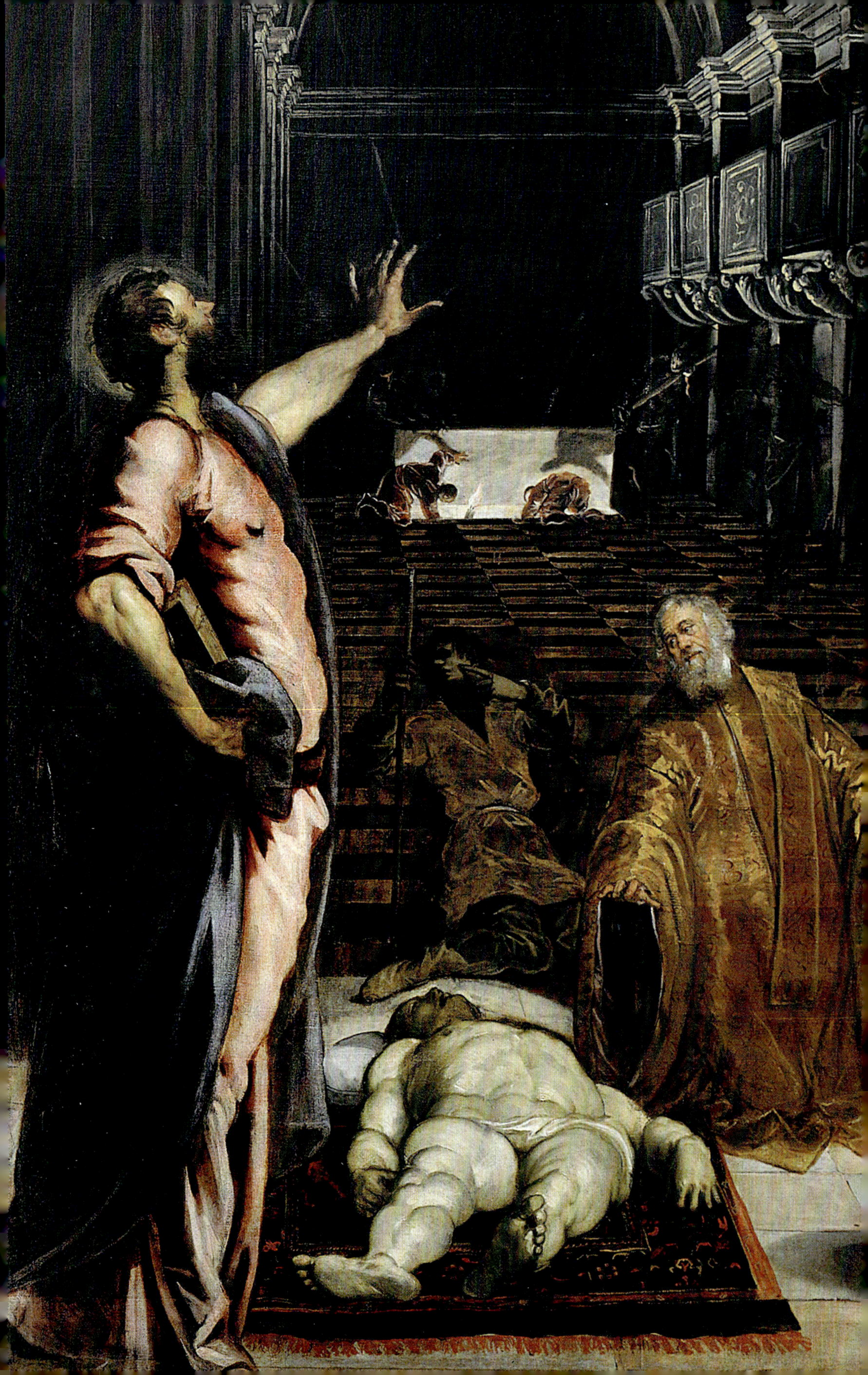

INTRODUCTION

Gabriele Matino, Cynthia Klestinec

THE TITLE OF THIS EXHIBITION, *Art, Faith and Medicine in Tintoretto's Venice*, highlights the potential insights and critical issues implicit in the combination of themes that are so distinct and yet closely interwoven with one another. If art, in the multiplicity of its forms and languages, has for centuries been used as an indispensable visual aid to the dissemination of religious and scientific ideas, the overlap and oscillation between the age-old systems of medical treatment and spiritual care is likewise a thread that runs through the whole of Christianity, its history, culture, and thought.

Ever since the origins of Christianity, the stories of miraculous healing related in the Gospels, the powers celebrated by the writers of the lives of the saints, and the legends about the miracles that have accompanied the transfer of relics from one place to another have given believers hope in cures supplementary to the ones offered by scientific medicine. To limit the result of such healing according to whether the treatment worked or not, however, is to underestimate the reach of divine intervention. Indeed, regardless of whether this kind of treatment might have a tangible impact on the ailing body, the manifestation of divine power had profound repercussions on both the patient restored to health and on the physician whose expertise had been so sensationally surpassed.

In the Gospels, Christ is portrayed as a healer: the blind, the deaf, the mute, lepers, the paralyzed, and the disabled of every kind all turned to him for succor. His powers offered early Christian writers and the Fathers of the Church the possibility of modeling, by analogy and through the metaphorical use of classical terminology, the figure of Christ the Doctor (*Christus medicus*): the almost spiritual Hippocrates, the true and only doctor, he who is both the doctor and the cure.[1] If at the root of the concept of Christ the Doctor lay the need to supplant the worship of healing deities like Aesculapius, Isis, Mithra, and Serapis, it is equally clear that the association between the figure of Christ and that of the physician can only be understood in a metaphorical sense. By representing Christ as a benevolent healer who took the affliction of others upon himself, doctors were offered an ethical and behavioral model to imitate,[2] while the sick were no longer perceived as targets of divine punishment but became instead emblems of Christ's sufferings. Thanks to this transformation in the status of the patient, the Christian doctor, who devoted himself to charity and to his fellow creatures, could trust, in turn, in a cure that would assuage the ills of his soul. In this way, medical treatment became a means

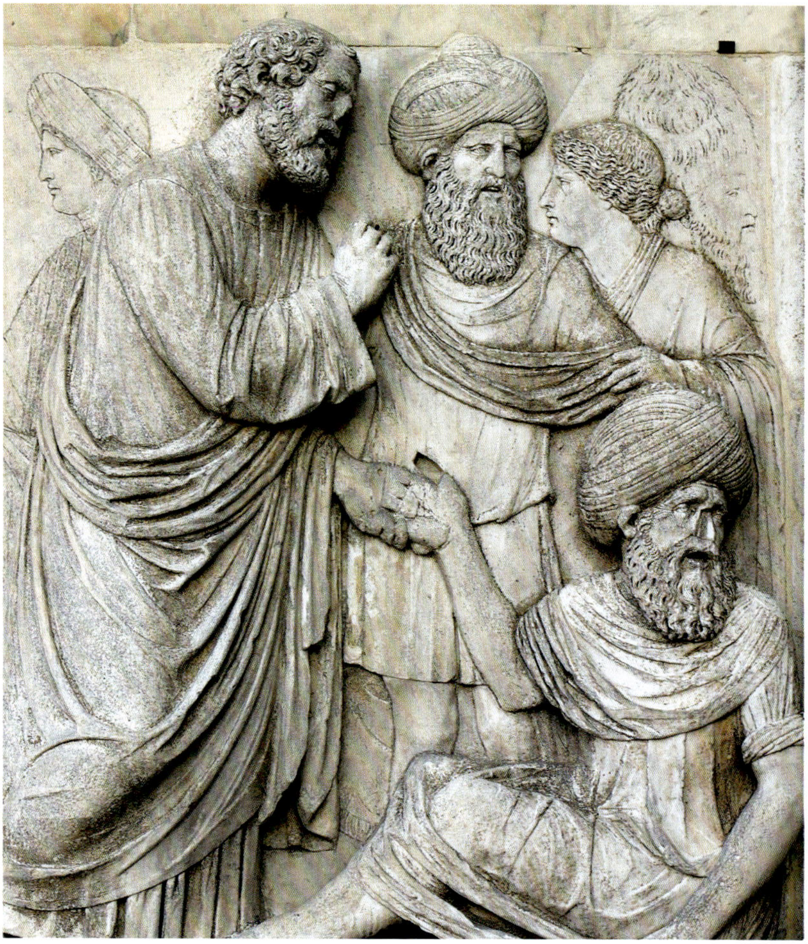

FIG. 1

of imitating the compassion of Christ the Doctor, who, to paraphrase Saint Cyprian, was made flesh in order to heal the wounds inflicted on humanity by the fall of Adam, neutralizing the venom of the serpent and prescribing his patients measures to avoid the illness's recrudescence.[3]

In the Middle Ages, this model of charity formed the basis of health care in the cities of northern and southern Europe. Venice's Scuole Grandi constitute a particularly representative example: these were lay confraternities that, though founded in the wake of the flagellant movement,[4] eventually turned into philanthropic organizations in which their original penitential vocation was replaced by a new mission to assist the most needy.[5] The main forms of charity promoted by the Scuole Grandi included the free provision of medical treatment and the establishment of almshouses. The Scuola Grande di San Marco was no exception. The reader may consult Paola Benussi's essay for an in-depth analysis of the phenomenon, and dwell, here, on the symbolic

FIG. 1
ANTONIO AND TULLIO LOMBARDO, *Healing of Anianus*, c. 1495. Venice, Scuola Grande di San Marco

significance of the medical assistance offered by the Scuola and on the use of art as the principal means of its promotion.

Saint Mark's biographers concur in describing him as a miracle-working saint. In Aquileia, the healing of the young noble Ataulf from leprosy fostered the cult of Saint Mark as doctor, and indeed some believe him to have belonged to the Alexandrine Therapeutae, a Jewish sect whose members were renowned for their asceticism and healing arts.[6] In Venice, the Evangelist's aid was sought for injuries, tumors, paralysis, blindness, possession, and the plague.[7] Mark was known for his curative powers in Alexandria as well: according to Procopius, the major Greek historian of Late Antiquity, pilgrims went to his tomb as if it were "the surgery of a doctor who dispensed treatment."[8] The miracle that caught the attention of the Scuola was that of the healing of Anianus, where the saint healed the injured hand of an Alexandrine cobbler with a salve made of saliva and earth. This episode was illustrated in a bas-relief carved by Antonio and Tullio Lombardo around 1495, and which was restored between 2000 and 2005, along with the entire architectural façade, with funding from Save Venice (fig. 1).[9] In displaying the miraculous healing on the front of the building, the brothers wanted to promote both the metaphorical value of Mark's act, itself modeled on the miracle of the healing of the man born blind, through which Christ cured the spiritual blindness of unbelievers (John 9: 1–41), and the charitable nature of the treatment offered by the Scuola to the poor, personified here by Anianus, whose pose calls to mind that of a beggar.[10] The miracle was also depicted by Giovanni Mansueti in a large canvas for the Sala dell'Albergo (after 1518; fig. 2), the place where the Scuola's officials used to meet. Just as the canvas reminded the brothers of the moral example they should be aspiring to, the words carved on the lintel of the room's doorway, *Ubi charitas et amor ibi deus est* (Where charity and love are, God is there), fixed in stone the principle on which the care of their fellow creatures ought to be founded.

Miraculous cures were attributed to Saint Mark even after his death: the miracles assigned to the presence of the saint's relics in Venice include healing cripples, resurrecting corpses, driving out evil spirits, and making it impossible for a cruel lord to have his servant's eyes put out as punishment for visiting the saint's resting place without his permission. At the Scuola, the depiction of Saint Mark's posthumous miracles was entrusted to Jacopo Tintoretto,[11] first in the famous *Miracle of the Slave* (c. 1548; fig. 4), and then in three large canvases commissioned in 1562 by Tommaso Giannotti Rangone (fig. 3, 6–7), the Scuola's director or Guardian Grande at the time, and a physician from Ravenna, whose life is described in greater detail in Sabrina Minuzzi's essay. In the paintings, Rangone appears next to the Evangelist, a privileged witness to the patron saint's miracles. However, the ostentatious way in which the images celebrated the exclusive bond between the doctor and the miracle-working saint was not well received by the Scuola's other

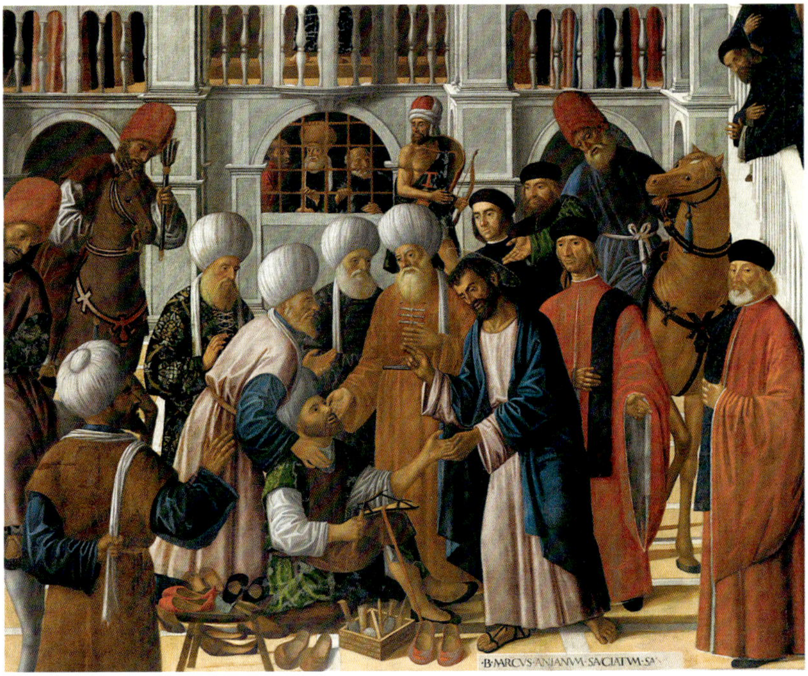

FIG. 2

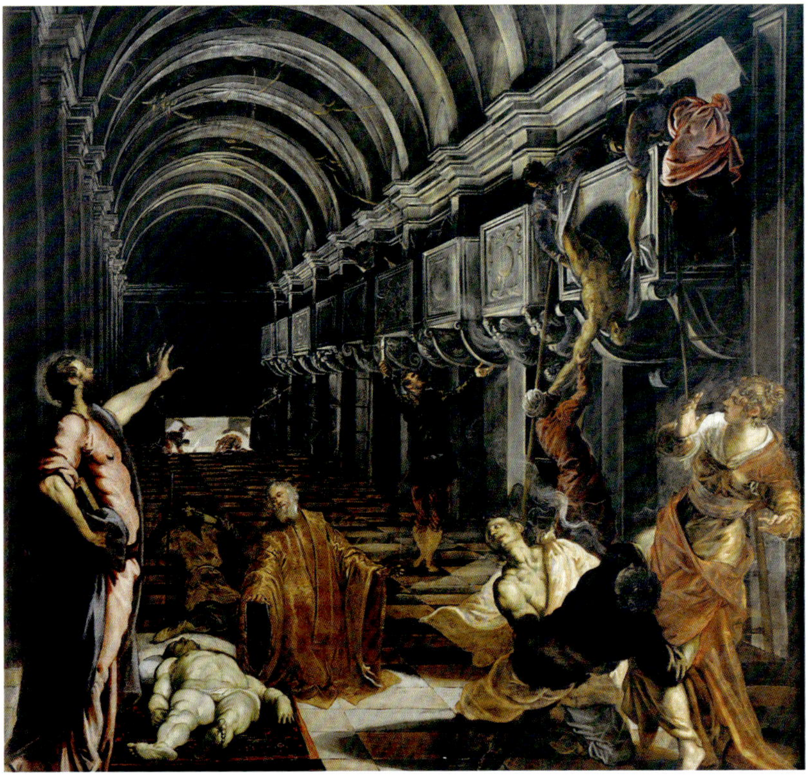

FIG. 3

FIG. 2
GIOVANNI MANSUETI, *Healing of Anianus*, after 1518. Venice, Gallerie dell'Accademia. Detail

FIG. 3
JACOPO TINTORETTO, *Miracles of Saint Mark* (also known as *Finding of the Body of Saint Mark*), c. 1566. Milan, Pinacoteca di Brera

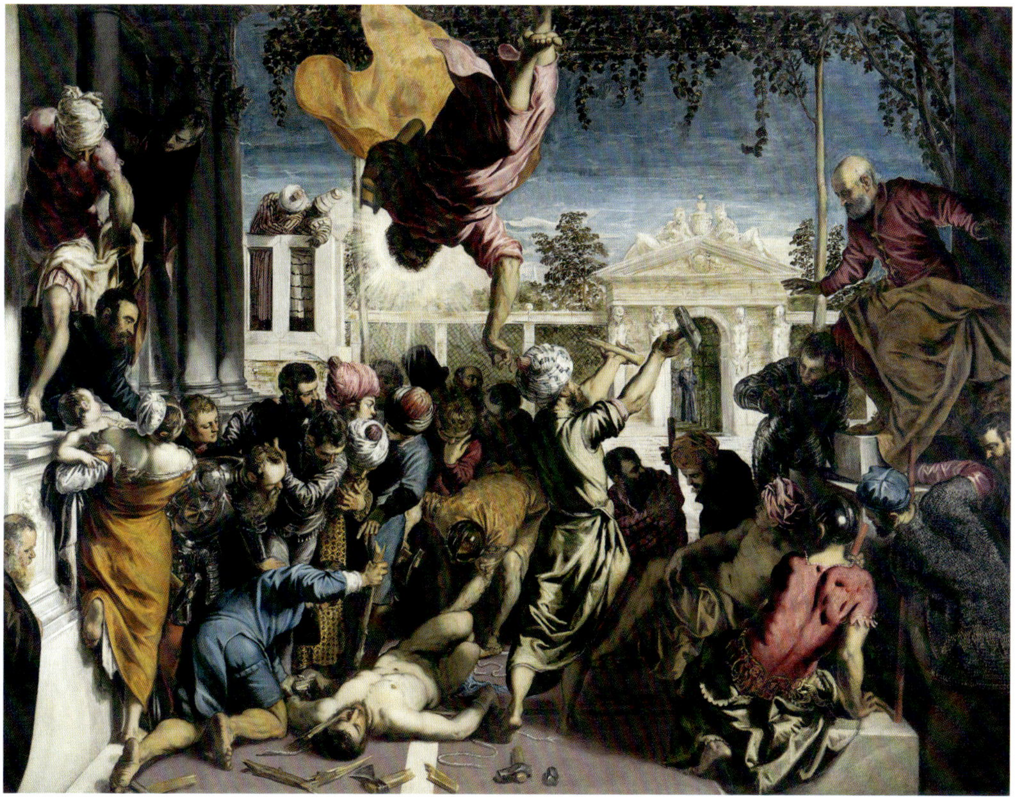

FIG. 4

officials, who tried, on several occasions, to have all depictions of Rangone removed from the pictures.[12] This was not the first time that Rangone's self-aggrandizing ambitions had met resistance, yet it is likely that there were deeper reasons behind the Scuola's protests in this case.

These reasons emerge more clearly if we compare Tintoretto's paintings with those of his son Domenico and Jacopo Palma il Giovane for the Scuola's chapel (c. 1587–92). These were restored in 2004–2014 with funding from Save Venice,[13] and have been put back in their original narrative order for this exhibition for the first time since their removal in 1806.[14] The cycle develops two of the constituent themes of the myth of Venice: the *Predestination* (*Praedestinatio*) and the *Transport of the Body of Saint Mark* (*Translatio*) to Venice.[15] The first is depicted in the *Dream of Saint Mark* (cat. 1), in which, during an overnight stay on the island of Rialto, the Evangelist experiences a vision in which an angel predicts his return to the lagoon following his martyrdom in Egypt. As for the *Transport of the Body of Saint Mark*, it was also depicted by Domenico in five canvases (two of which have been lost) that showed the voyage of the saint's relics to Venice and its arrival in the city, focusing on the ultimate fulfillment of divine will (cat. 2–3, 5). It is

FIG. 4
JACOPO TINTORETTO, *The Miracle of the Slave*, c. 1548. Venice, Gallerie dell'Accademia

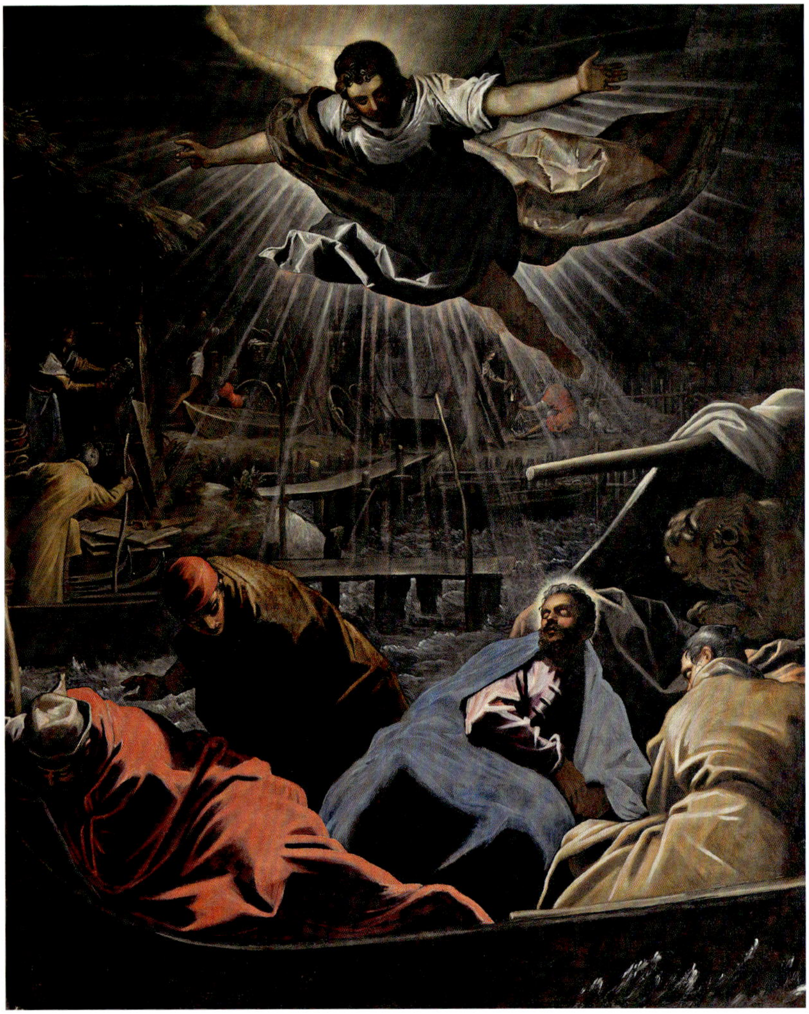

CAT. 1

obvious that Rangone's desire for the limelight would have been regarded as inappropriate in the context of a cycle of paintings intended to celebrate the inclusion of Venice within God's plan of salvation.

The chapel's altarpiece (cat. 6) supports this hypothesis by privileging the glorification of the Venetian Republic over the celebration of specific individuals. For a better understanding of the clients' intentions, it is helpful to look at the sketches submitted to the Scuola by Domenico Tintoretto (1612) and Palma il Giovane (1614). In Domenico Tintoretto's sketches, Saint Mark receives the pastoral staff and miter in the presence of the Guardian Grande, who is portrayed as closely involved in the event, and who restricts its effects to the bounds of the Scuola (The British Museum, London, inv. 1097,0717.21). Palma's sketch, which eventually won him the commission, shifts the

CAT. 1
DOMENICO TINTORETTO,
Dream of Saint Mark,
c. 1587–90

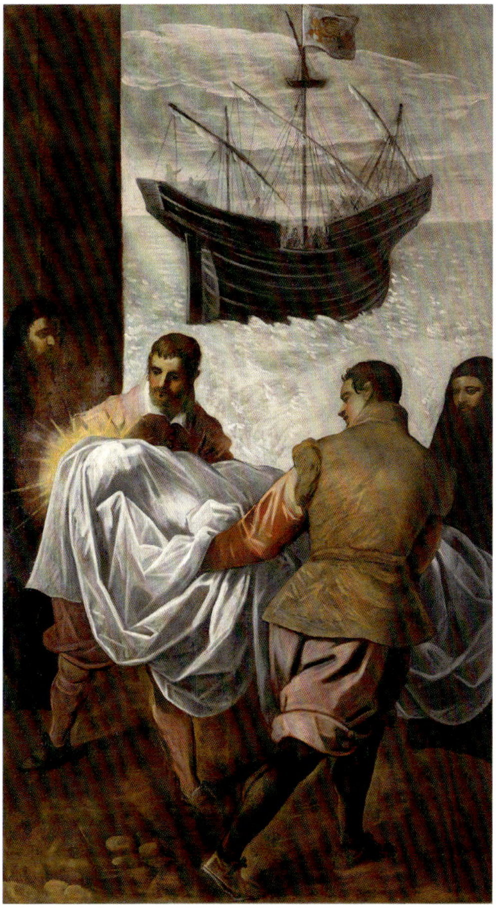

CAT. 3

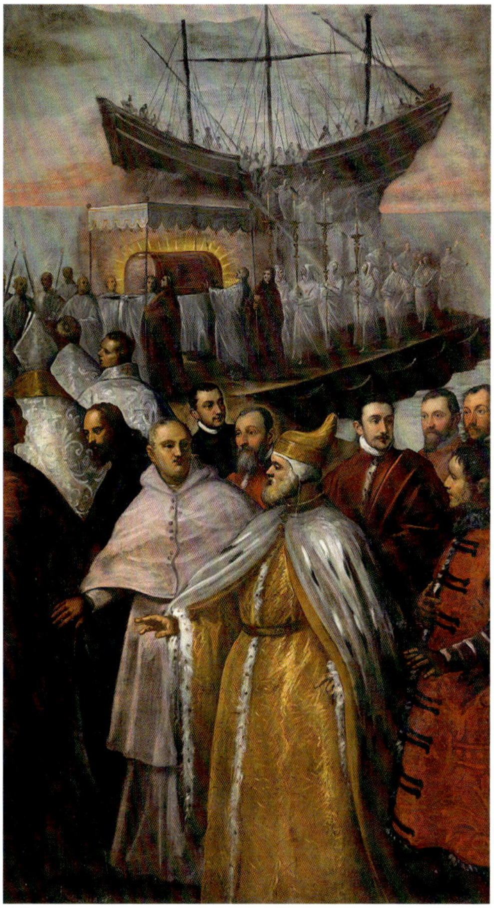

CAT. 5

scene outside the confines of the brotherhood through the exclusion of the Guardian Grande — a request specified in the conditions for the competition for the altarpiece (1614)[16] — and the relocation of the Evangelist's "glory" above his city (fig. 5). The transfer of the martyr's attributes from Saint Mark to Venice implied the extension of his power over the entire Venetian Republic, here extolled in its political (the Palazzo Ducale), religious (the Basilica di San Marco), and imperial (the Bucintoro, the doge's barge) prerogatives. It is no accident that, in the painting, Saint Peter and Saint Paul are placed at Saint Mark's feet, as an expression of Venice's pre-eminence over the Church, especially at a time when the consequences of the 1606–07 diplomatic dispute between Venice and the Holy See (also known as Venetian Interdict) were still being felt. While this is not the place to discuss the reasons behind the dispute, it is worth recalling the support that the Scuole Grandi gave to the Venetian cause, both in reassuring the population over the threat of

CAT. 3
DOMENICO TINTORETTO, *Transport of the Body of Saint Mark to the Venetian Ship*, c. 1590

CAT. 5
DOMENICO TINTORETTO, *Arrival of the Body of Saint Mark in Venice*, c. 1590–92

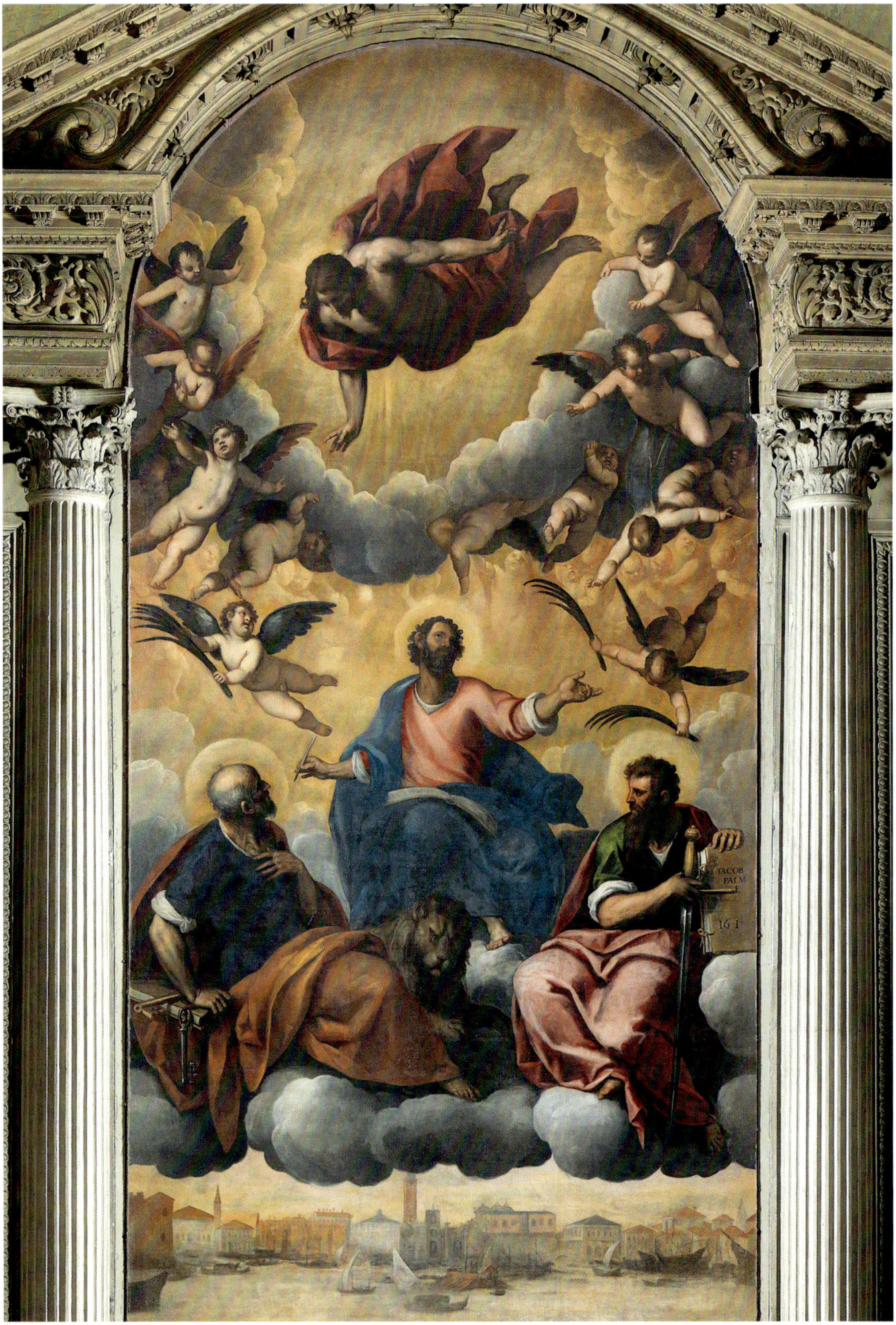

CAT. 6

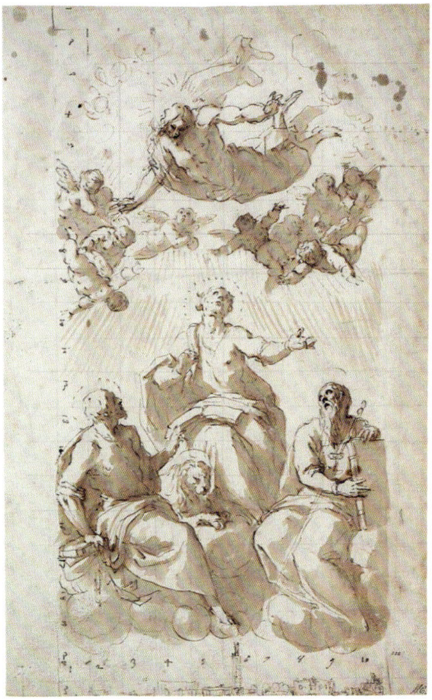

FIG. 5

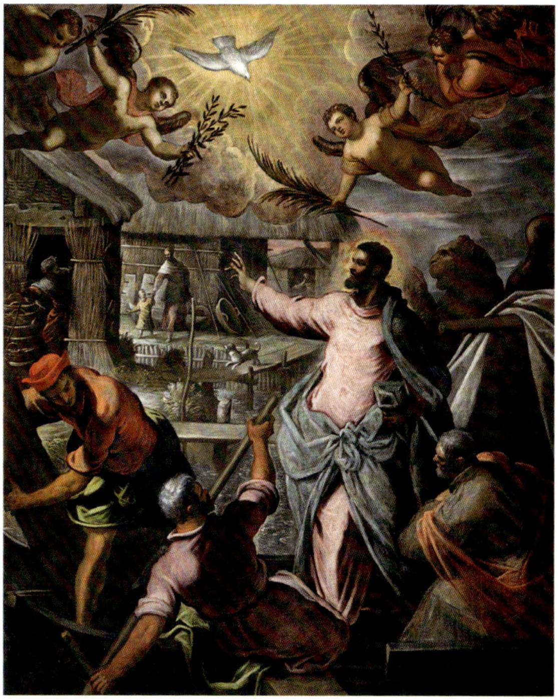

CAT. 2

excommunication and in disseminating Venice's doctrines regarding the separation of Church and State.[17] By reminding viewers of the *Predestination* and the *Transfer of Saint Mark's Body* to Venice, and therefore also the prominent role Saint Mark played in Venice's founding, the chapel's paintings also renewed Venice's claim to sovereignty.

CAT. 6
JACOPO PALMA IL GIOVANE, *Saint Mark in Glory with Saints Peter and Paul*, 1614–15

FIG. 5
JACOPO PALMA IL GIOVANE, sketch for *Saint Mark in Glory with Saints Peter and Paul*, 1614. London, Victoria & Albert Museum

CAT. 2
DOMENICO TINTORETTO, *Saint Mark Blessing the Venetian Islands*, c. 1587–90. Venice, Scuola Grande di San Marco

The iconographic program reached its conclusion with the *Miracle of the Ring of Saint Mark*,[18] a work by Domenico Tintoretto that was originally located in the vicinity of the chapel and which, taking its cue from the *Appearance* (*Apparitio*) or *Discovery* (*Inventio*) of the Evangelist's body, completed the trilogy of the myth of Saint Mark (cat. 4). The painting depicts a miracle that occurred at the time of the rediscovery of the saint's body (June 25, 1094), when it emerged from a pillar in the Basilica di San Marco giving off a fragrant odor — from which we have the appellative "Saint Mark of rosewater" — in demonstration of the incorruptibility of his flesh and in prefiguration of victory over death. Tradition has it that one of those present was Domenico (also known as Zuane or Zuandomenico) Dolfin, who, in order to receive the gift of the Evangelist's ring, made a vow to share its curative properties with all of the saint's devotees (cat. 15). After staying in the hands of the Dolfin family for centuries, the ring was sold by Lorenzo Dolfin to the Scuola for 100 ducats in 1509. From then on, every June 25 the Scuola took part in civic

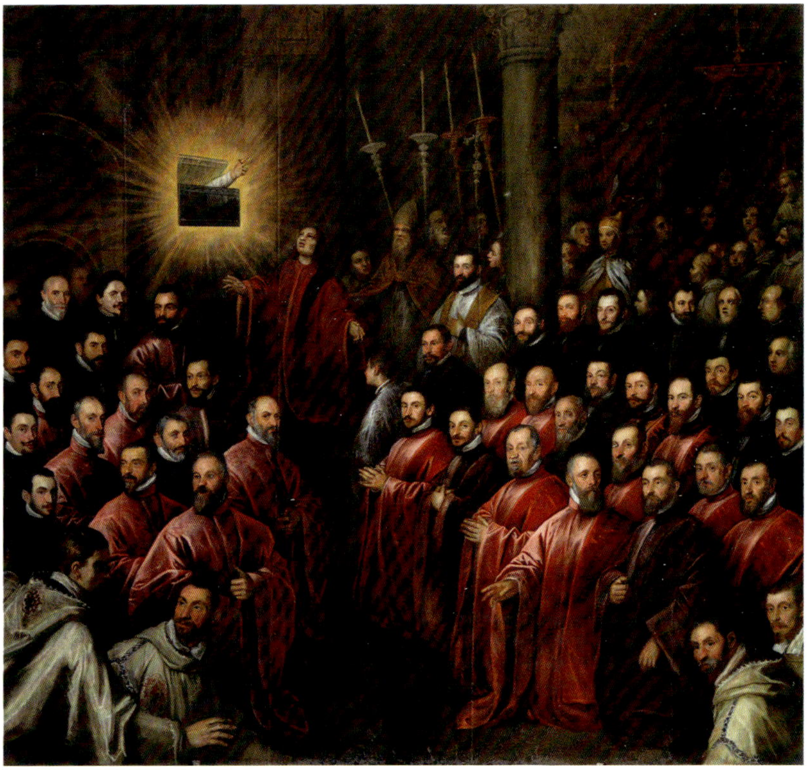

CAT. 4

and religious commemorations of the *Appearance*, bringing the ring to the Basilica di San Marco, where the sick waited to be cured.[19] Unfortunately, in 1575 the Scuola was robbed of the precious relic,[20] forcing the brothers to commission a painting in which the apparition of Saint Mark memorialized, and thus perpetuated, their special relationship with their patron saint.

By associating the gift of the ring with portraits of the Scuola's officials, the painting identified the confraternity as the privileged repository of the saint's compassion, the inspiration and ultimate aim of the cures the brothers offered. Moreover, in accordance with the will of the Scuola's founding fathers, who had established it in honor of the "State of the City of Venice,"[21] the painting shows the brothers as they take Dolfin's vow upon themselves, extending the miraculous power of the Evangelist to the entire city. Finally, considered in light of the themes developed in the whole cycle of paintings, the *Miracle of the Ring of Saint Mark* made it possible to reconcile the mythical time of *Predestination*, *Transfer*, and *Appearance* with the historical time of Saint Mark's posthumous miracles, thereby reconfirming the central role Venice played in God's designs.

G.M.

CAT. 4
DOMENICO TINTORETTO, *Miracle of the Ring of Saint Mark*, end of the sixteenth century

CAT. 15
Saint Mark Gives His Ring to Domenico Dolfin, in *Passio Sancti Marci...*, fourteenth century

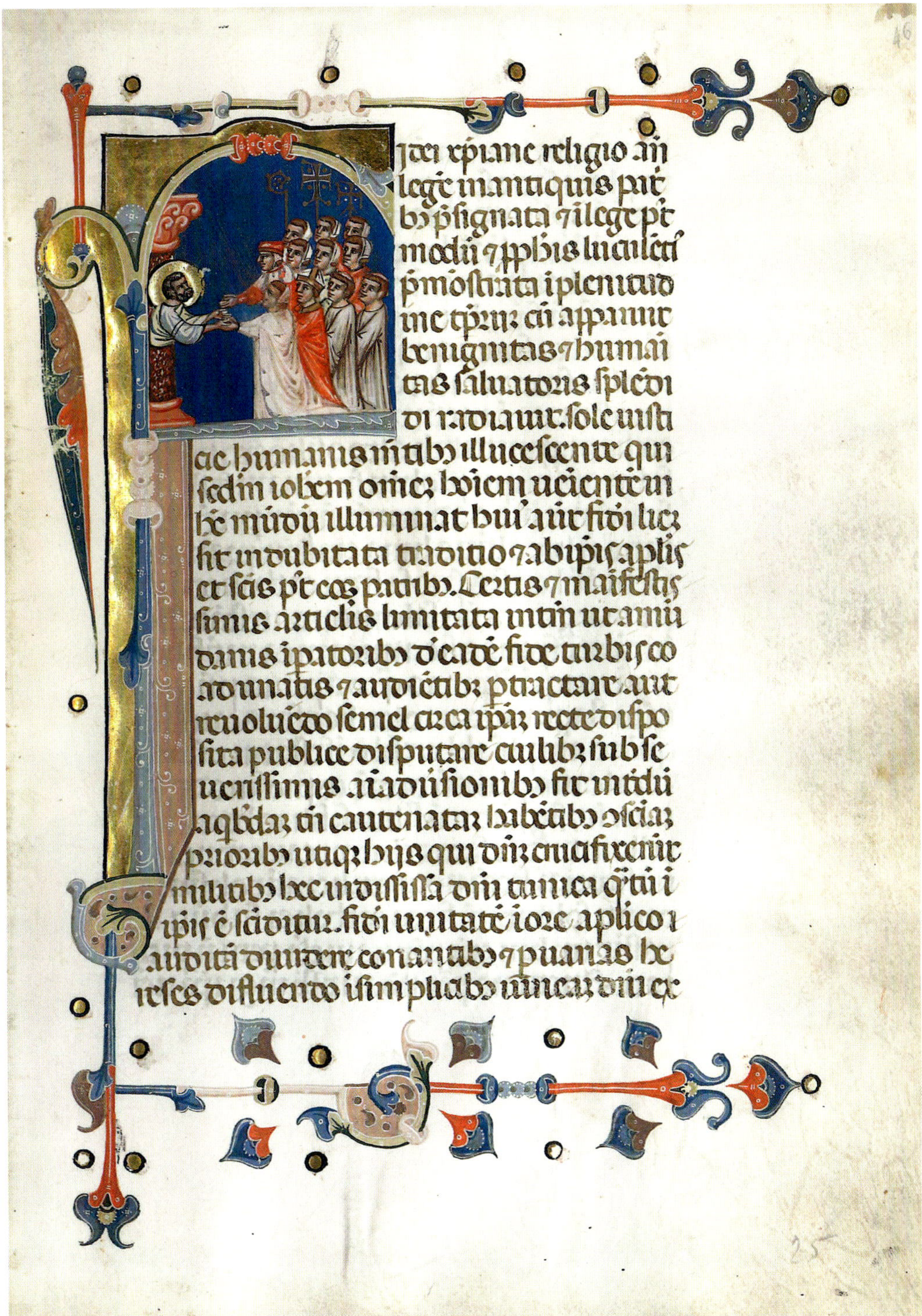

CAT. 15

IT WAS NOT only the pictorial tradition that spoke of the significance of medicine and of spiritual and bodily health, but also its key historical actors. Tommaso Rangone, the physician described in Sabrina Minuzzi's essay, extended the range of his interests beyond the practice of medicine. He engaged the wider world of Venice with its prolific printing presses and its variegated artistic culture, amassing a collection of books and other artifacts that testify to his interests, curiosities, and commitments. In addition to the humanist topics on display in his collection and his deep interest in paintings, Rangone included several works that focused on the plague. The latter affliction, as Michelle Laughran explores in her essay, compelled a range of responses from the Venetian government, including the establishment of a health board (on which practitioners such as Rangone served) and specific policies regarding quarantine and the efforts of charitable groups. These developments coincided with a deeper and more widespread questioning of the society about the relationship between spiritual and bodily health, the practice of prophecy and astrological medicine, and what physicians called *medicina mentis et corporis* (medicine of the mind and body). In her essay, Jennifer Gear explores the different kinds of depictions and references to plague in the city's visual culture of the time.

In addition to his interest in the plague and both traditional and novel diagnostics, Rangone shared his peers' fascination with the study of human anatomy — a fascination also cultivated by medical practitioners and, as discussed by Gabriele Matino in his essay, by artists like Jacopo and Domenico Tintoretto. Rangone's collection included texts on human anatomy and the practice of dissection. Since at least the time of Galen (c. 130–210 AD), medical practitioners had recognized the need for a basic understanding of human anatomy and the potential for its study to unlock some of the secrets of the human body. At universities across Europe, special theaters were built for the purposes of studying the anatomy of human and animal bodies. As Cynthia Klestinec explains in her essay, inside these theaters professors of anatomy would read passages from ancient sources while an *ostensor* would point to the part of the body under discussion, so that a dissector could carry out the dissection (cat. 33). Thus the anatomical theater was, for a time, firmly centered on the figure of the professor and his books.[22] Although anatomy would seem to demand a more direct encounter between the viewer and the corpse, we should remember that even today there are various kinds of mediation in the anatomy lab, such as diagrams and more naturalistic images obtained via computer simulation. While these provide indirect rather than direct access to the body, they serve pedagogical functions that have counterparts in the sixteenth century, where images helped to clarify structures and the relations between them.[23]

This academic tradition of anatomy complemented the more practical considerations of medical practitioners. If we travel from sixteenth-century

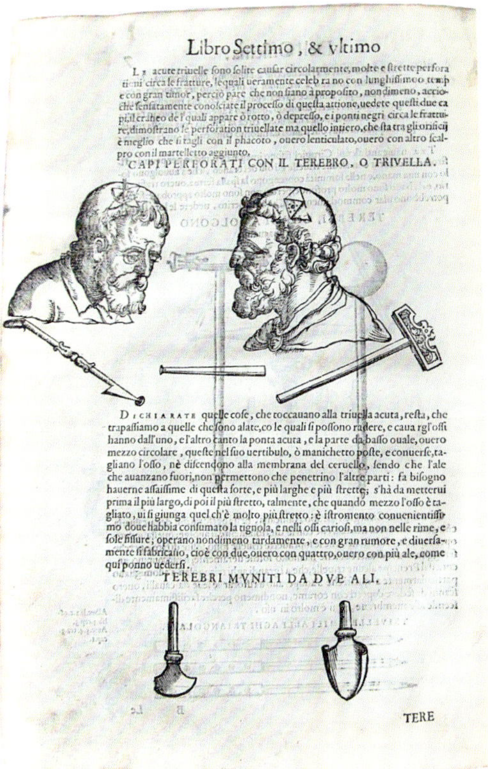

CAT. 49

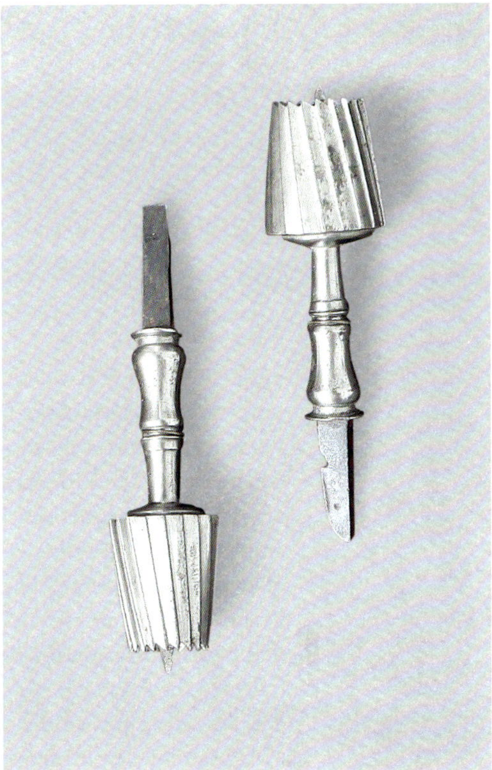

CAT. 73

CAT. 49
GIOVANNI ANDREA DALLA CROCE, *Cirugia vniuersale e perfetta di tutte le parti pertinenti all'ottimo chirurgo...*, Venice, 1583

CAT. 73
Cranium drill and bits, sixteenth century

Padua and its university to Venice and its health care institutions, we encounter another conversation about anatomy. In sixteenth-century Venice, elite medical practitioners emphasized the importance of attending anatomy demonstrations, even for barbers. Attendance at these events became a desirable criterion for appointments to government positions. Anatomy was politicized even as it began to establish itself as an important aspect of elite medical culture in Renaissance Venice.

This increasingly articulate and extended conversation was directed, in part, by the hierarchy of medical practitioners. As Paolo Savoia explains in his essay, surgeons could occupy a broad range of positions within public health institutions. In places like France, they were seen as similar to barbers and set apart from physicians, while in Italy, especially near universities, surgeons could receive academic training and benefit from advantageous collaborations with physicians. In Venice there was a vibrant tradition of university-trained surgeons: they formed their own College of Surgery, published in Latin and Italian, and practiced alongside physicians such as Rangone.[24] Surgeons and physicians shared not only patients, but also a perspective on medicine and culture that was truly interdisciplinary, even visionary. This perspective included an interest in instruments and the notion of the hand as an extension of the intellect's rational faculties.

Descriptions of the ideal surgeon at the time also included his ability to make instruments, not just use them. Indeed, the treatise on surgery written by Venetian surgeon Giovanni Andrea dalla Croce (cat. 49) includes illustrations of instruments that can be seen in the exhibition, next to actual instruments, which have been attributed to Croce himself (cat. 73). These two sets of instruments, the ones in the illustrations and the ones in real life, show how these books could serve multiple audiences and roles: not only did Croce's text describe the ideal surgeon and present him as well-educated in the ancient tradition of medicine, but it may also have served to advertise instrument-makers' craft or even to provide guides for the instruments' construction. The production and use of anatomical and surgical texts entailed a range of artisans associated with image-making, as Ilaria Andreoli emphasizes in her essay. These material artifacts reflect the collaboration of anatomists and surgeons with artisans, such as the one who used color in the oil paintings associated with Hieronymus Fabricius's oil paintings to distinguish anatomical structures. The forms of these anatomical figures reflected the era's iconographic trends and tastes. Iulius Caesar Casserius's anatomy text shows cadavers in various states of dissection, who reveal their own anatomies by lifting flaps of skin. The conceit was an elaboration of the dictum "know thyself" and connected these works to an older tradition of "flap" anatomies as well as to the pictorial innovations of the age.[25]

C.K.

NOTES

1 R. Arbesmann, "The Concept of 'Christus Medicus' in St. Augustine," *Traditio*, 10 (1954), 1–28.

2 G.B. Fergren, *Medicine and Health Care in Early Christianity* (Baltimore: Johns Hopkins University Press, 2009).

3 Arbesmann 1954, 7.

4 See Paola Benussi's essay in this volume.

5 B. Pullan, *Rich and Poor in Renaissance Venice: the Social Institutions of a Catholic State, to 1620* (Oxford: Blackwell 1971).

6 G. Pressacco, "Marco 'christianus et medicus,'" in *San Marco: aspetti storici e agiografici, atti del convegno internazionale di studi (Venezia, 26–29 aprile 1994)*, ed. A. Niero (Venice, 1996), 647–84.

7 *San Marco Evangelista. Opere d'arte dalle chiese di Venezia*, ed. A. Manno (Venice: Grafiche Veneziane, 1995), catalogue for the exhibition (Venice, Church of San Bartolomeo, February 18-May 31, 1995).

8 Ibid.

9 M. Conn and D. Rosand, eds., *Save Venice Inc: Four Decades of Restoration in Venice* (New York-Venice: Save Venice Inc., 2011), 160–65.

10 L. Buonanno, "A Charitable 'Façade'? The Sculptural Decoration of the Scuola Grande di San Marco," *Confraternitas*, 21 (2010), 6–16.

11 R. Battaglia, "'I miracoli di San Marco' di Jacopo Tintoretto nella Sala Capitolare," in *La Scuola Grande di San Marco a Venezia*, Mirabilia Italiae series, ed. G. Ortalli and S. Settis, (Modena: Franco Cosimo Panini, 2017), 135–54.

12 See "Chronology."

13 Conn and Rosand 2011, 160–65.

14 See "Chronology."

15 D. Rosand, *Myths of Venice: The Figuration of a State* (Chapel Hill-London: University of North Carolina Press, 2001).

16 See "Chronology."

17 Pullan 1971.

18 G. Matino, "Per una nuova lettura dell'*Apparitio* di Domenico Tintoretto: il *Miraculum de anulo beati Marci*," in *La Scuola Grande di San Marco a Venezia*, eds. Ortalli and Settis, 161–64, 270–71.

19 P. Fortini Brown, "Honor and Necessity: The Dynamics of Patronage in the Confraternities of Renaissance Venice," in *Studi Veneziani*, 14 (1987), 179–212.

20 Archivio di Stato di Venzia (henceforth ASVe), Scuola Grande di San Marco (henceforth *SGSM*), b. 22, cc. 220r-228r; ASVe, *Consiglio dei Dieci*, "Deliberazioni criminali," Registri, 12, cc. 83v-84r.

21 ASVe, *SGSM*, b. 216.

22 Andrea Carlino, *La fabbrica del corpo: Libri e dissezione nel Rinascimento* (Turin: Einaudi, 1994), published in English as *Books of the Body: Anatomical Ritual and Renaissance Learning* (Chicago: University of Chicago Press, 1999); and Giuseppe Ongaro, "La medicina dello studio di Padova e nel Veneto," in *Storia della cultura veneta. Dal primo Quattrocento al Concilio di Trento*, Vol. 3 (Vicenza: Neri Pozza, 1981), 76–134.

23 On the subject of contemporary anatomy laboratories, see *Anatomies: De Vésale au Virtuel*, ed. V. Barras (Lausanne: Éditions BHMS, 2014). For a historical account of how images were produced and used in Renaissance anatomy (as well as in botany), see Sachiko Kusukawa, *Picturing the Book of Nature: Image, Text, and Argument in Sixteenth-Century Human Anatomy and Medical Botany* (Chicago: University of Chicago Press, 2012).

24 Richard Palmer, "Physicians and Surgeons in Sixteenth-Century Venice," *Medical History*, 23 (1979), 451–60.

25 Andrea Carlino, *Paper Bodies: A Catalogue of Anatomical Fugitive Sheets, 1538–1687* (London: Wellcome Institute for the History of Medicine, 1999).

¶ Libro da compagnia o vero di fraternita di batturi novamẽte stãpato: ⁊ diligẽtemẽte corecto cõ molte aditione a laude de dio ⁊ de la gloriosa virgine maria: ⁊ de li devoti christiani. Et historiato.

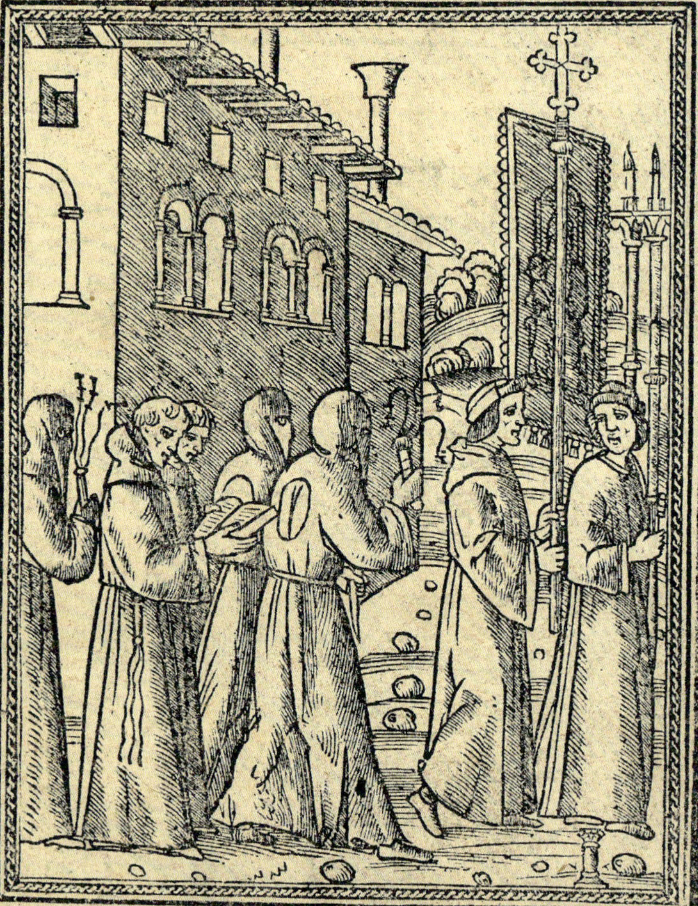

INVESTMENT IN CHARITY: THE WELFARE ACTIVITIES OF THE SCUOLA GRANDE DI SAN MARCO IN THE SIXTEENTH CENTURY

Paola Benussi

THE SCUOLA GRANDE DI SAN MARCO was established as a confraternity of flagellants some time before 1261 at the church of Santa Croce, in the Venetian *sestiere* (district) of the same name. In 1438, the Scuola moved to a location next to the central convent of Santi Giovanni e Paolo. Its seat would remain there — in a building reconstructed in the form we see today following the disastrous fire of 1485 — until the abolition of all confraternities decreed in 1806 by the legislation of the Napoleonic Kingdom of Italy.[1] Its centuries of activity should be seen in the context of the institutional development of all Venetian Scuole Grandi, each of whom went through a similar evolution.

Emerging in Venice in the wake of the rapid spread of the flagellant movement throughout Italy from 1260 onward, the *scuole dei battuti*, as they were known, gave the impetuous religious fervor of the movement an organized form, channeling it into orderly and permanent activities of worship, penitence, and charity. The structure of the lay confraternity, combining forms of communal devotion and mutual assistance, provided the organizational framework that these new associations required in order to turn into enduring institutions. The Venetian *schole verberatorum* (flagellant confraternities) were subjected to state control from the very start, like every other association. This shows that their importance was immediately recognized, although it was not until 1467 that they were given the official designation of Scuole Grandi (*scholae magnae*) to distinguish them from the city's other, smaller confraternities (*scholae communes*). Thanks to the bequests they attracted from the mid-fourteenth century onward, the Scuole Grandi were able to combine their devotional practices — centering, for the collective, on public processions (cat. 57), and, for the individual brothers, on preparations for a good death and rites of intercession — with charitable and welfare activities. Over the course of the fifteenth century, charity became increasingly important, and the Scuole Grandi took on the character of charitable institutions, with the aim of containing and providing a response to urban poverty, even though they limited their efforts to their own members.[2] This transformation entailed a radical change in the social hierarchy within the Scuola. While it was open to members of all the city's classes, the original equality of all members gave way to a subdivision into two distinct, wealth-based segments: the richer members, for whom the management of the association was reserved,[3] gave alms to the poorer ones, who in turn became entirely responsible for the religious and penitential practices carried out for the spiritual benefit of the entire confraternity.[4]

CAT. 57
Libro da compagnia o vero di fraternita di battuti..., Venice, 1518, 22 September

In the case of the Scuola Grande di San Marco, this evolution was clearly reflected in the words chosen to conclude the record of the transfer of its headquarters in the Scuola's notarial register: these words invoked the Trinity, and specifically they asked the Virgin Mary and Saint Mark, the Father, Son, and Holy Spirit to "look after it and defend it from every misfortune and help and multiply the possessions of the confraternity for the good and benefit and aid of the poor and give grace and life to our purpose."[5] By recognizing the polarity between charity to the poor and salvation of the soul as the core of the material and spiritual benefits offered to the brothers, the emphasis was placed on elements that diverged from the expiatory and communitarian approach of the early days. This last was instead effectively represented by the iconography of the two miniatures (cat. 16) set at the beginning of the *mariegola* (statute book) of the mid-fourteenth century.[6] Here, opposite the scene in which the brothers, dressed in processional tunics (*cape*), attend the ceremony of admission of a novice,[7] was placed an image of the *Flagellation* to represent the salvific function of self-flagellation practiced publicly by the flagellants, in what was the key feature of the confraternity.

The material assistance offered by the Scuole to their poor members was divided, as we will see, into a well-structured range of types of economic support. All the Scuole Grandi provided many of their brothers, in different quantities and proportions, not only with alms (donations of money or in kind intended to meet immediate and contingent needs), but also with more systematic and targeted forms of aid, such as *grazie* given to poor girls to be used as dowries, free housing (*amore Dei*, "for the love of God"), admission to the *ospizio* (as the hospital was called at the time) for anyone who, unable to work, could not rely on family support, and medical treatment and medicines for those unable to afford the expense.[8]

In 1590 the Scuola Grande di San Marco, one of the least prosperous Scuole Grandi at the time, owing to a drastic reduction in the yield of the sovereign bonds in which the greater part of its capital was invested, possessed twenty-six houses that it provided free of charge to the poor — a much smaller amount of real estate than was owned by the other Scuole Grandi[9] — and reserved almost half the sums allocated for charitable activities for alms (49.23%) and about a third for dowries (33.25%), with the rest split more or less equally between expenditure on the hospital (9.44%) and medical care (8.07%). The proportions changed considerably over the course of the next two decades, settling on new priorities that saw a very large rise in the share spent on dowries (50.94%), to the detriment mainly of alms (35.48%), but also of hospital (6.79%) and health care expenditures (6.79%). Although they were probably in part the result of external factors like taxation, these variations show that the main types of assistance, alongside alms-giving, took the form of dowries and housing.

As far as alms were concerned, the Scuola Grande di San Marco made a special collection of money ("universal charity") that was divided each year

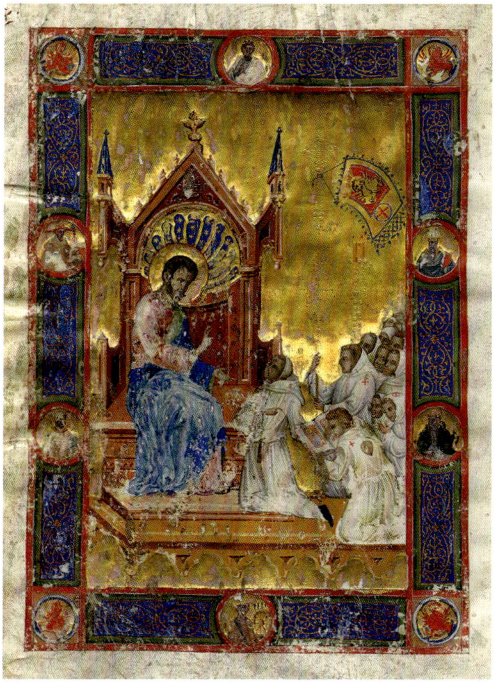

CAT. 16 (A)

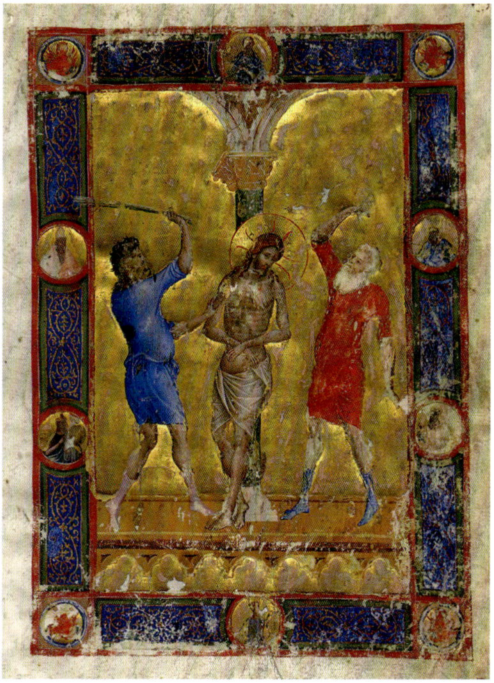

CAT. 16 (B)

among indigent members.[10] The need for the control and rationalization of contributions led to the distribution of coupons for the collection of alms, which were later replaced by *tessere*: these consisted of a sort of bronze medal bearing the symbol of the Scuola and, often, a legend (*pietas* or *charitas*) referring to the token's function (cat. 69–70).[11] In addition to this institutionalized charity to which all the brothers contributed, the Scuola distributed the income from the *commissarie* or trust funds bequeathed to it in the manner laid down by the testators. One of the most substantial of these was the annuity, in flour and wine, established by Tommaso Morosini in 1532.[12]

The custom of making bequests to help girls get married and setting up more lasting foundations for the same purpose had been widespread in Venice since the Middle Ages. It was seen as a form of both material and spiritual charity since, by allowing young women to wed in a regular manner, it countered the danger of social marginalization in situations that would also have put the health of their souls at risk. For a sense of the phenomenon's scale, it is worth pointing out that in 1581 Francesco Sansovino declared that the six Scuole Grandi "marry off each year [...] over 1500 maidens with the proceeds from bequests."[13] The Scuola Grande di San Marco was the first to permanently allocate a substantial sum to fund these young girls or *novizze*. As early as 1392, it invested the sum of 12,000 ducats in the *Camera degli Imprestidi* (Chamber of Loans), and the resulting returns were used to fund twelve dowries of thirty

CAT. 16
PAOLO VENEZIANO (attrib.), *Illumination from the* mariegola *of the Scuola Grande di San Marco. Initiation of a Novice in the Presence of the Brethren and Saint Mark* (A), *Flagellation of Christ* (B), mid-fourteenth century

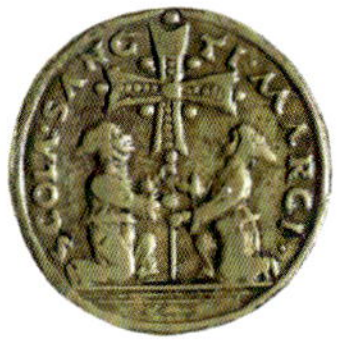

CAT. 69

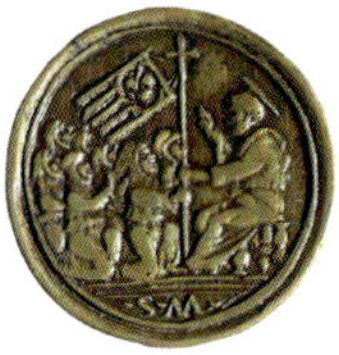

CAT. 70

ducats each annually.[14] The decision may have been prompted by the example set just a few years earlier by the brother Ludovico Buora, whose will (August 12, 1387) had established a trust fund, managed by the Scuola itself, to provide dowries for twelve sailors' daughters, a third of whom were to be chosen from among the daughters of members of the Scuola.[15] However, the Buora legacy was just the first[16] of a total of thirty-eight bequests out of 135 made between the middle of the fourteenth century and the end of the seventeenth to benefit poor young women.[17] The dowries were assigned to girls aged at least thirteen, on the basis of a system that combined an assessment of merit with the casting of lots, a procedure also used for other types of benefits in which the demand greatly exceeded the possibility of meeting it.[18] The young women presented themselves at the Scuola, and its officials (the *banca*) examined their candidacies, weighing up the requisites of material necessity and morality. Those considered worthy, and who had obtained two thirds of the votes of the *banca*, were included in the drawing of lots fixed for January 21, the feast of Saint Agnes.[19] On that occasion each girl drew a *segno*, a small rectangle of silk on which was written either *patientia* (patience) or *gratia* (granted), indicating the outcome of the lottery. The maiden whose request had been granted obtained the right to receive one of the dowries on offer, although it was not paid out until after the wedding. The procedure just described is the reason for the preservation in the Scuola's archives of numerous receipts for the payment of the sum, issued by the husbands of the young lottery winners.[20] In some cases they still have, rolled up in the parchment along with the declaration of the parish priest who had conducted the wedding, the precious dotal *grazia* along with an inscription in gilt letters, the symbol of the Scuola, and the year of the lottery, a tangible memento of the confraternity's charity (cat. 25). It was also still possible for girls who had drawn the *segno* marked *patientia* to obtain a dowry from the Scuola, as the members of the *banca* and *zonta* (auxiliary governing board), at least in the sixteenth century, offered money from their own pockets for the benefit of these young women. According to data gathered by Brian Pullan, in the decade between 1550 and 1560 the Scuola Grande di San Marco funded dowries for a total of 459 *donzelle* (maidens), at a gross outlay of 8,063 ducats.[21]

CAT. 69, 70
Badge of the Scuola Grande di San Marco, sixteenth century

As has already been suggested, another area of assistance that had an incisive social impact was that of the housing provided *gratis et amore Dei*. In

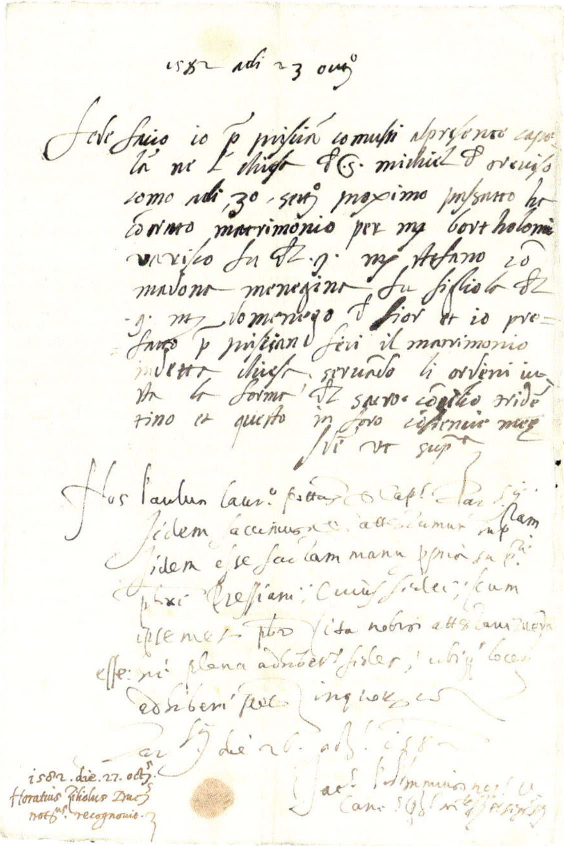

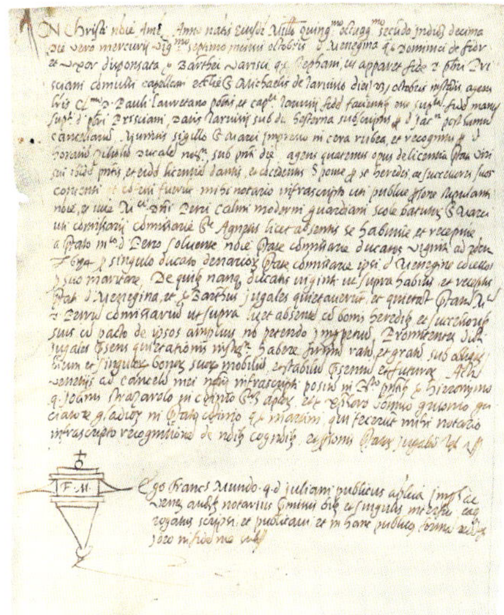

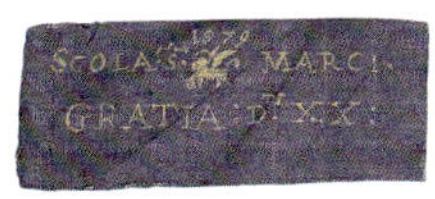

CAT. 25

this sector, too, the assignment to brothers in need depended on an assessment of the candidates' merit, which took into account both economic and moral criteria.[22] From an analysis of the properties still declared in the eighteenth century,[23] it seems possible to conclude that most of the *amore Dei* homes were located in two residential complexes, both of which had been left to the Scuola by members in their wills. The first was a bequest from Pietro Arbosani, a "wealthy man and noble merchant"[24] who, in his will dated January 24, 1425, had left his houses in the districts of Santa Croce and San Silvestro for the benefit of poor brothers.[25] The houses in Santa Croce, located in the same parish as the seat of the Scuola at the time, faced the *fondamenta* (a street along a canal) of the monastery of the same name and were entered from a porch and courtyard that from then on were named after Saint Mark (cat. 8).[26] The second group of dwellings, in this case built from scratch on an undeveloped site in Santa Maria Maggiore, in the ward of the Angelo Raffaele, in an urban setting characterized by similar initiatives undertaken by the Scuola Grande di San Rocco and the Procurators of Saint Mark, had an identical effect on the city's

CAT. 25
Receipt given to Guardian Grande Tommaso (Giannotti Rangone)...,
1569, February 3

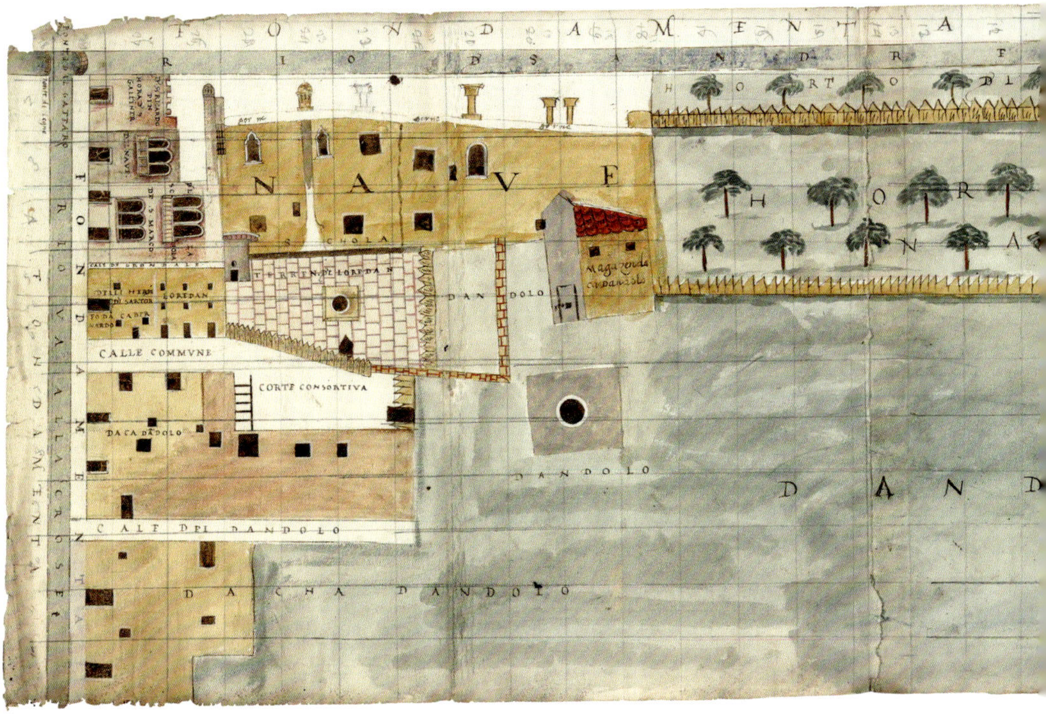

CAT. 8

toponymy. Thanks to the legacy of Pietro Olivieri, who in his will of October 25, 1515, left a large sum to the Scuola Grande di San Marco expressly to be used for the construction of homes for brothers "from good families" and "that above all have children,"[27] a courtyard surrounded by twenty-four houses, all still in existence, was built between 1529 and 1542.[28]

Like other Scuole Grandi,[29] that of San Marco set up a hospital, perhaps as early as the third quarter of the fourteenth century. In 1348, in the earliest will we know of containing dispositions in favor of the Scuola, Martin de Griffon from San Silvestro established that, after the death of his heirs, four *case da sarzenti* (low-rent houses) at Quintavalle (San Pietro di Castello) should go to the Scuola Grande di San Marco, on the condition that they be turned into hospitals for ailing brothers — a condition that, however, was never met.[30] In any case, it can be assumed that, on that date, a hospital run by the confraternity did not yet exist. Once again, it is a will that indicates the *terminus ante quem* for the hospital's establishment: on February 10, 1377, Iacomello da Riva bequeathed the annuity of a *miro*[31] of oil to the poor admitted to the Scuola's hospital.[32] It must have only been founded very recently, as an article of the *mariegola* makes reference to the license granted in 1374 to the Guardian Grande — as a result of a decision taken by the doge and his councilors, the heads of the Quarantia and the Maggior Consiglio — to "lodge eight of our poor brothers, who will be

CAT. 8
Scuola houses in the sestiere of Santa Croce, sixteenth century

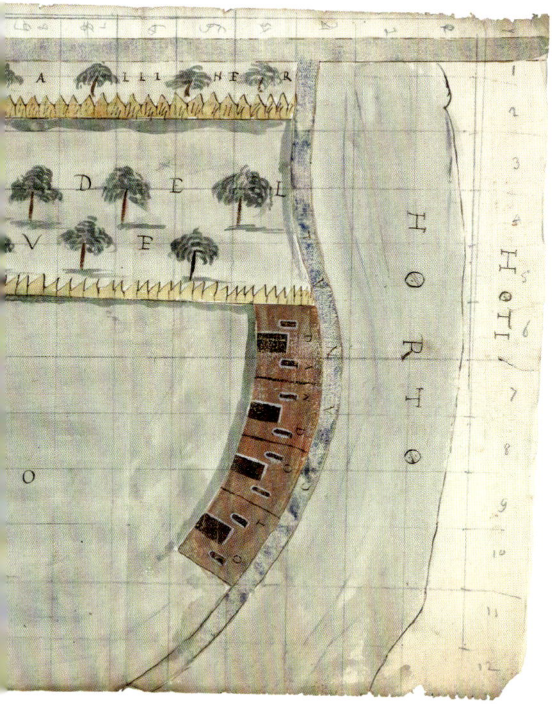

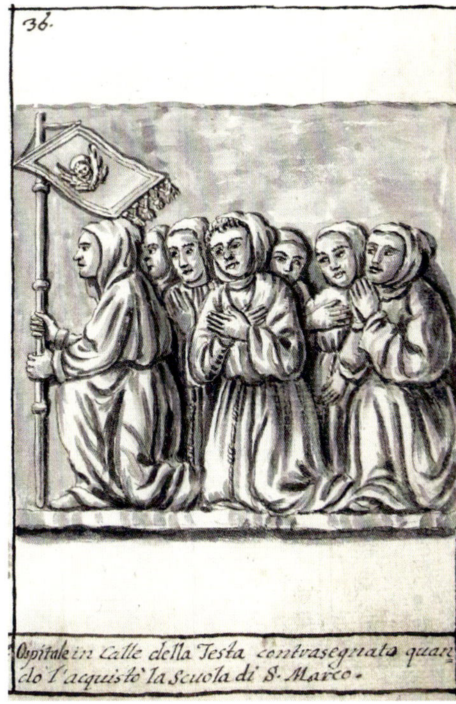
36.
Ospitale in Calle della Testa contrasegnata quan
do l'acquistò la Scuola di S. Marco.

CAT. 14

recognized as the most needy, in one of our houses in Santa Croce supplied with eight beds."[33] Over the course of several decades, the *ospizio*, originally housed in a building adjoining the seat of the Scuola, drew the attention of other testators, who left part of their estate to the small institution.[34]

In 1473, after the confraternity's transfer to Santi Giovanni e Paolo, the *capitolo* (chapter general) decided that the hospital should move as well.[35] A decade later, a suitable plot of land was found, but then the initiative was put on hold, perhaps as a result of the fire of 1485. In 1491, however, one of the brothers, Lunardo Corradin, gave the Scuola his *casa da statio* (house for rental) in Calle della Testa, in the parish of Santa Maria Nova, under the condition that it be converted into a hospital after his death, which occurred in 1495.[36] Once again things turned out to be more complicated than envisaged, but by the beginning of the sixteenth century, the new structure was finally in operation (cat. 14).[37] Initially intended to house six, and then eight patients, managed by a prior and looked after by a *massara* (housekeeper), the hospital's capacity was reduced for economic reasons in the sixteenth century. We know what the situation was after the middle of the century after the visit paid by the Guardian Grande at the time, Tommaso Rangone (1562),[38] but the definitive *regolatione* (regulations) were established with the resolution of the *banca* and *zonta* on June 20, 1591, when its statute was systematically reformulated. At the

CAT. 14
GIOVANNI GREVEMBROCH,
Varie venete curiosità sacre e profane, 1755

time, there were only three poor patients, but their number was raised to five (and reduced to four soon after); the prior was appointed for life, but subject to reconfirmation every four years on the basis of an assessment of his work.[39] The brothers admitted to the *ospizio* were not allowed to spend the night outside the structure without special permission, and in 1615 they were also required to wear "a Saint Mark painted on white cloth," a public declaration of the fact that they were being maintained at the expense of the confraternity.[40]

Just as in the other Scuole Grandi, at San Marco doctors were accepted free of charge and exempted from the self-flagellation, in exchange for the treatment of sick brothers.[41] Between 1480 and 1549, the *mariegola* listed sixty *miedexi de fixicha* (physicians) and eighty-one *miedexi de piaga* (surgeons).[42] At the beginning of the sixteenth century, regulations were tightened to avoid free-loading and to limit the service to members who would otherwise be unable to afford it: specifically, from 1511 onward, doctors could only examine patients with the permission of the Guardian Grande or his deputy, who would take it upon themselves to verify whether examination was necessary.[43] However, it was around the middle of the century, between 1541 and 1544, that the way the Scuola provided health care truly changed, since, from then on, it was to be dispensed by two physicians appointed by the confraternity and paid an annual fee of twelve ducats. In 1552, they were joined by a surgeon on a salary of four ducats, soon raised to ten.[44] In the sixteenth century, physicians who were affiliated with the Scuola[45], either as benefactors or as members, included one of the most sought-after Venetian practitioners of his time, Nicolò Massa (1489–1569), who acquired renown and wealth through his skill in diagnosing and treating a number of different diseases.[46] An author of scientific works and an influential member of the College of Physicians whose opinion was sought even from abroad, Massa decided that after the death of his heirs and the executors of his will a trust fund comprising the whole of his estate should be set up. Its management would be entirely entrusted to the Scuola, on the condition that one third of the income be distributed to "poor and needy" brothers and another third to the "wretched poor" of the city, while the remaining third could be reserved for maintenance expenses and payment of the taxes levied on the trust fund.[47]

Whether as the result of decisions taken by the governing bodies or the inclinations of individual brothers, the full range of the Scuola Grande di San Marco's charitable activities in the sixteenth century, in all their different forms, constituted the material dimension in which the confraternity's principles of Christian charity found tangible expression, in a distinctive balance of aspiration to eternal salvation and respect of the social order.

NOTES

1 For the history of the Scuola and a general picture of the activity of the Venetian Scuole Grandi, see E. Orlando, "La Scuola Grande di San Marco a Venezia. La storia e le fonti," in *La Scuola Grande di San Marco a Venezia*, *Mirabilia Italiae* series, ed. G. Ortalli and S. Settis (Modena: Franco Cosimo Panini, 2017), 13–31 (with bibliography).

2 B. Pullan, "Poveri, mendicanti e vagabondi (secoli XIV-XVII)," in *Storia d'Italia. Annali 1: Dal feudalesimo al capitalismo* (Turin: Einaudi, 1978), 989–90; ibid., *La politica sociale della Repubblica di Venezia 1500-1620*, Vols. 1–2 (Rome: Il Veltro, 1982); id., "The Scuole Grandi of Venice: some further thoughts," in ibid., *Poverty and Charity: Europe, Italy, Venice, 1400-1700* (Aldershot: Ashgate, 1994), 273–301. See also D. Romano, "L'assistenza e la beneficenza," in *Storia di Venezia. Vol. 5: Il Rinascimento. Società ed economia*, ed. U. Tucci and A. Tenenti (Rome: Istituto della Enciclopedia Italiana, 1996), 355–406.

3 From 1410 the executive posts of the Scuole Grandi were reserved by law for native-born citizens and, on a more limited basis, for those who had been granted citizenship (Pullan 1978, Vol. 1, 113–49).

4 Ibid., 74–113.

5 ASVe, *SGSM*, reg. 16 bis, p. 11, April 25, 1438, cited in Orlando 2017, 16–18.

6 L. Humphrey, *La miniatura per le confraternite e le arti veneziane. Mariegole dal 1260 al 1460* (Verona: Cierre Edizioni 2015), 191–98.

7 G. Matino, "Osservare la Regola. Usi e funzioni delle miniature trecentesche della *Mariegola* della Scuola Grande di San Marco," in *Costantinopoli e Venezia. Fondazioni bizantine di carità e Scuola Grande di San Marco*, ed. F. Lauritzen (Rome, in press).

8 Pullan 1978, Vol. 1, 178–210, from which the figures given in the following paragraph are also taken.

9 Ibid., 203. At around the same time (1581), the Scuole Grandi di San Rocco, di San Giovanni Evangelista and della Misericordia were able to offer their members forty-four, seventy-six and sixty free lodgings, respectively.

10 Orlando 2017, 24.

11 G. Majer, "Le tessere delle scuole religiose di Venezia," *Rivista italiana di numismatica e scienze affini*, 2 (38), third series (1925), 17–40. For a broader picture see W.J. Courtenay, "The King and the Leaden Coin: the Economic Background of 'Sine Qua Non' Causality," *Traditio*, 28 (1972), 185–209, in particular 196–97, and ibid., "Token Coinage and the Administration of Poor Relief during the Late Middle Ages," *The Journal of Interdisciplinary History*, 3 (2), (1972), 275–95.

12 G. Matino, "Flour, Wine and Atonement: Domenico Morosini's *Annual* and the Poor Brothers of the Scuola Grande di San Marco," in *"Ebbi fame e mi deste da mangiare." Luoghi, principi e funzione della* charitas *veneziana 1260–1806, atti della giornata di studi (Venezia, Scuola Grande di San Marco, 18 settembre 2015)*, ed. G. Matino and N. Gietz (Modena: Franco Cosimo Panini, 2018), 89–103. See also I. Cecchini, "Il pane e i poveri. Carità presso la Scuola Grande di San Marco in età moderna," ibid., 75–88.

13 F. Sansovino, *Venetia città nobilissima et singolare* (Venice, 1581), f. 99v. In "The Council of Ten and the Scuole Grandi in Early Renaissance Venice," *Studi Veneziani*, n.s., 18 (1989), 51: 15–66. W.B. Wurthmann calculates that in the fifteenth century the four Scuole Grandi in existence at that time were able to provide dowries for at least fifty girls each year.

14 Orlando 2017, 25; P. Fortini Brown, "Le scuole," in *Storia di Venezia. Vol. 5 Il Rinascimento. Società ed economia*, 307–54, in particular 344.

15 ASVe, *Notarile, Testamenti*, b. 557,

unnumbered coupon and register of documents cc. 49r-50v. ASVe, *SGSM*, b. 216, dated March 24, 1392.

16 In reality, the oldest will with dispositions to the benefit of the Scuola Grande di San Marco, that of the bricklayer Martin de Griffon, dated April 5, 1348, to which we will return later, already provided for the funding of dowries as an alternative should it not be possible to fulfill the wishes expressed by the testator in the first instance (ASVe, *SGSM*, reg. 11, on that date).

17 ASVe, *SGSM*, regs. 11 and 14.

18 The number of female applicants in the sixteenth century has been estimated at 130–140 per year (Pullan 1978, Vol. 2, 714).

19 The day was later moved to the following Sunday: Orlando 2017, 25.

20 ASVe, *SGSM*, bb. 71, 72, 267.

21 Pullan 1978, Vol. 2, 713. There were 334 girls who were aided (6205 ducats) from the returns on the trust funds, 112 (1721 ducats) with voluntary contributions from the *banca* and *zonta*, and thirteen (137 ducats) on petition.

22 B. Pullan, "Abitazioni al servizio dei poveri nella Repubblica di Venezia," in *Dietro i palazzi. Tre secoli di architettura minore a Venezia 1492-1803*, ed. G. Gianighian and P. Pavanini (Venice: Arsenale 1984), 39–43, exhibition catalogue (Venice, Scuola Grande di San Giovanni Evangelista, 29 September-9 December 2012); G. Guidarelli, "Le Scuole grandi veneziane nel XV e XVI secolo: reti assistenziali, patrimoni immobiliari e strategie di governo," in *Mélanges de l'École française de Rome – Moyen Âge*, 123, 1 (2011), 59–81; ibid., "Pietre come pane. L'architettura e la politica assistenziale delle Scuole grandi veneziane," in Matino and Gietz 2018, 63–73.

23 In 1720 the Scuola Grande di San Marco declared to the Inquisitori e revisori sopra le Scuole Grandi that it had thirty-nine houses to be granted *amore Dei*: fourteen at Santa Croce (Arbosani bequest), twenty-four in contrada dell'Angelo Raffaele (Olivieri bequest) and one in Santa Margherita (Pantaleone Cattaneo bequest, June 17, 1450), see: ASVe, *SGSM*, b. 126, fasc. marked IV E 18, c. 5; for Cattaneo's will: ibid., reg. 11, at that date; Fortini Brown 1996, 343.

24 See previous note. E.A. Cicogna, *Delle inscrizioni veneziane* (Venice: Orlandelli, 1824), Vol. 1, 150–51, no. 44.

25 ASVe, *SGSM*, reg. 11, at that date.

26 The houses no longer exist. Cicogna (1824) mentions the plaque placed above the entrance to the porch after its restoration in 1548.

27 ASVe, *SGSM*, reg. 11, at that date.

28 P. Fortini Brown, *Private Lives in Renaissance Venice: Art, Architecture, and the Family* (New Haven-London: Yale University Press, 2004), 203–05. From the second decade of the eighteenth century only twenty of the homes were granted *amore Dei*, as the other four were rented out to fund the maintenance of the residential complex (ASVe, *SGSM*, b. 144).

29 Pullan (1978, Vol. 2, 722–723) records, in addition to that of the Scuola Grande di San Marco, the *ospizi* of the Scuole Grandi di San Giovanni Evangelista (San Geremia and San Stin), della Misericordia (San Marcilian), and della Carità (San Trovaso).

30 ASVe, *SGSM*, reg. 11, at that date. Although the Scuola took possession of the houses around 1474–75, due to what seems to have been a misunderstanding of the will's provisions, its governors did not fulfill the obligation, but rented them out, only realizing their error in 1676 (ASVe, *SGSM*, b. 164, fasc. "Martin de Griffon").

31 Venetian unit of measurement for oil corresponding to 15.7898 liters. See A. Martini, *Manuale di metrologia ossia misure, pesi e monete in uso attualmente e anticamente presso tutti i popoli* (Turin: E. Loescher, 1883; anast. reprint, Rome: E.R.A., 1976), 818.

32 ASVe, *SGSM*, reg. 11, at that date.

33 ASVe, *SGSM*, b. 149, fasc. "Carte circa l'ospedale della veneranda Scola di San Marco evangelista," c. 2.

34 On December 29, 1386, Vecellio Premarin, formerly Raniero from San Polo, left a homestead of two meadows at Biancade, in the province of Treviso, to the hospital of the Scuola "for the assistance of the poor"; on August 29, 1398, Pantaleone Partidor from Santa Fosca established that the rent paid by the tenants of his house be set aside for ten years to buy clothing for the hospital's poor; on August 8, 1416, Piero da Vigna, formerly Alban, a *calafato* (caulker) from San Pietro di Castello, earmarked the rent from a house in his district for the hospital's poor; finally, on June 14, 1474, Giacomo Alemante instructed the Scuola to invest his estate in *imprestidi* (loans), setting aside a quarter to fund the building and ornamentation of the Scuola and its hospital (ASVe, *SGSM*, reg. 11, at those dates).

35 Orlando 2017, 18–19.

36 ASVe, *SGSM*, b. 155, fasc. "Veneranda Scuola di San Marco per la commissaria del quondam Lunardo Corradin quondam Corrado," perg. no. 5 and b. 156, fasc. marked G. On the location of the now demolished building, see F. Semi, *Gli "Ospizi" di Venezia* (Venice: Istituzioni di Ricovero e di Educazione, 1983), 205.

37 Orlando 2017, 19.

38 Cecchini 2018, 83–84.

39 ASVe, *SGSM*, reg. 8, cc. 238v-239v.

40 ASVe, *SGSM*, b. 156, dossier marked G, c. 53.

41 ASVe, *SGSM*, reg. 8, c. 347r. See E. Orlando 2017, 19, 22; A. Porro e L. Lorusso, "La Scuola come istituzione e l'assistenza sanitaria," in *La Scuola Grande di San Marco a Venezia*, ed. Ortalli and Settis, 33–42.

42 ASVe, *SGSM*, reg. 4. The categories into which members of the Scuola were divided were, in order of rank: priests, patricians ("nobles of the Council"), the two classes of physician, the brothers exempt "from self-flagellation," and the ones subject to it.

43 ASVe, *SGSM*, reg. 8, c. 347v.

44 Ibid., cc. 347r-v, 351r.

45 From the Scuola's own sources, they included Giovanni Coronelli (will of July 29, 1447: ASVe, *SGSM*, reg. 11, at that date, and b. 154), Giovanni Domenico del Negro (will of May 29, 1515: ibid., reg. 11 at that date), and Nicolò Rinio (will of April 21, 1604: ibid., reg. 11, at that date). All three men are also known from other documents.

46 R. Palmer, "Nicolò Massa, His Family and His Fortune," *Medical History*, XXV (1981), 385–410, and L. Roscioni, "Massa, Nicolò," in *Dizionario biografico degli italiani* (Rome: Istituto della Enciclopedia Italiana, 2008), Vol. 71, 674–77.

47 L.R. Lind, *Studies in Pre-Vesalian Anatomy: Biography, Translations, Documents* (Philadelphia: American Philosophical Society, 1975), 325–32.

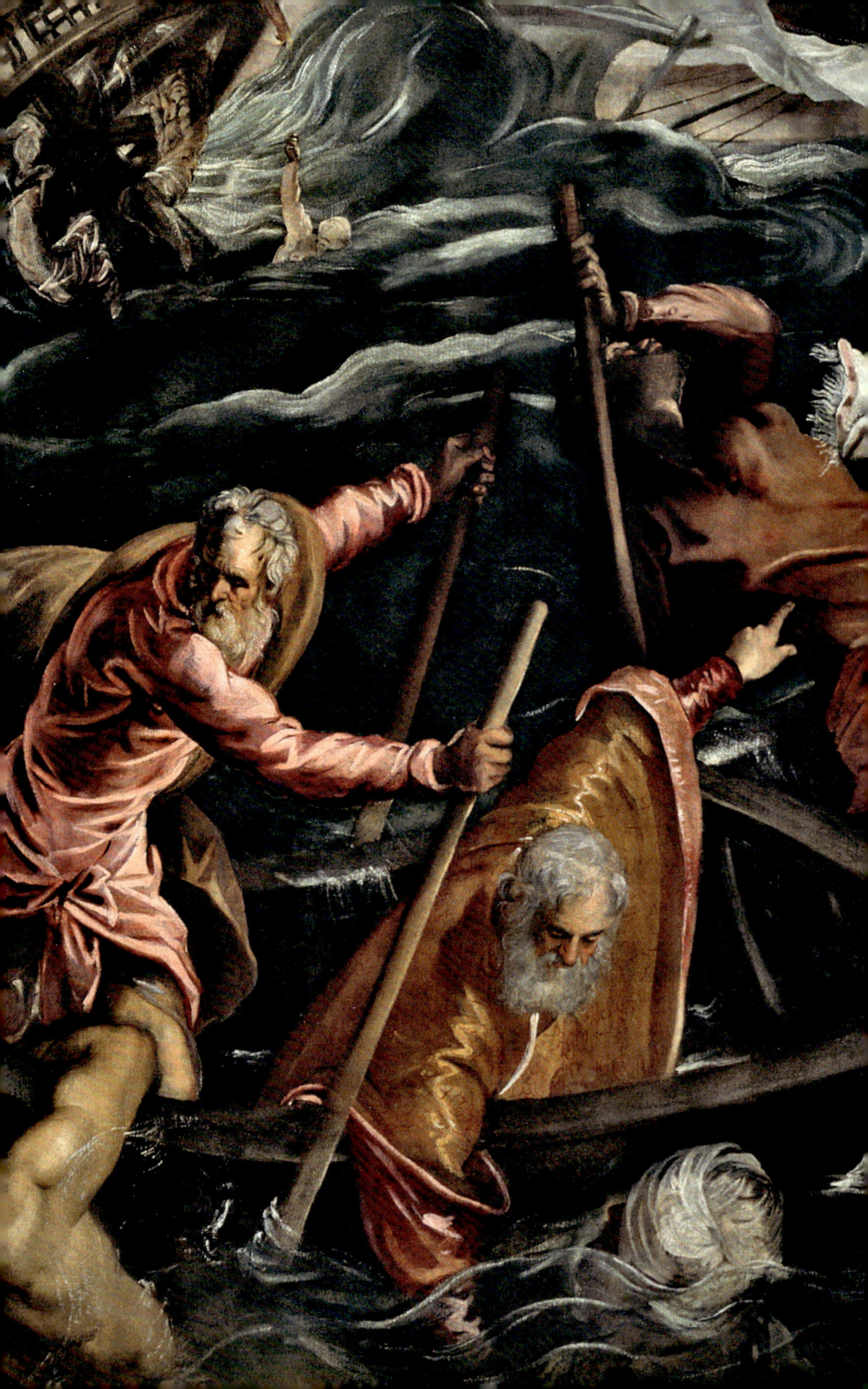

TOMMASO GIANNOTTI RANGONE: A LIFE MODELED ON BOOKS AND (NOT JUST MEDICAL) ART

Sabrina Minuzzi

ONE OF THE most representative figures of sixteenth-century Venetian medicine, with regard both to its practice and to the embedding of the profession in the social fabric, was undoubtedly Tommaso Giannotti Rangone, who is well known thanks to the marked narcissism that induced him to leave indelible traces of himself all over the city and his era. Tommaso was active on several fronts: he published books that disseminated his medical knowledge; he had medals struck and statues sculpted to immortalize his effigy among symbols of the art of medicine; and, finally, he commissioned paintings of sacred subjects that celebrated his devotion to Saint Mark. He dedicated his books to popes, doges, and doges' wives, and he placed statues and pictures in key places of worship, making religious faith the background and the ideal setting for his image as a physician.

Tommaso was born in Ravenna on August 18, 1493, to a family of small means.[1] After an initial study of the classics, as a result of which he assumed the title of *Philologus* beginning in 1513, he took courses in philosophy and medicine in Rome, Ferrara, and Bologna, interspersed with intervals of teaching to fund his studies. In Bologna he defended his thesis on medicine on March 13, 1513, and graduated in *artibus et medicina* on August 21, 1516.[2] From the end of 1516 to 1520 he taught sophistry at La Sapienza in Rome, astrology in Bologna, and mathematics and astrology at the University of Padua. However, he soon gave up teaching to enter the service of Count Guido Rangone in the capacity of physician and astrologer at his small court in Modena, at that time a papal stronghold. During the 1520s he accompanied the count on his military campaigns. Writing prognostications for the count and popes brought him to the attention of the courts, but these activities also entangled him in the controversy over judicial astrology, seen by detractors as an insidious and effective way of interpreting political moods and manipulating collective fears.[3] Then, while maintaining excellent relations with the count, who even allowed him to adopt his own surname, in the early 1530s the forty-year-old Tommaso moved to Venice to devote himself to the practice of medicine, "not caring to exercise the profession of astrology in Vinegia [Venice]."[4] Indeed, while natural astrology was an established subject at universities, undifferentiated even in name from what we call astronomy today, in the late fifteenth century the debate over judicial astrology, which interpreted the influence of the planets on human destiny in a deterministic manner, had flared up again, eventually prompting the

Church to condemn it as heresy.[5] Tommaso was quick to perceive the decline of astrological prediction and ceased to practice it.

TOMMASO'S MEDICAL AND SCIENTIFIC PRODUCTION

After moving to Venice, Tommaso devoted himself to his medical practice with such success that he was able to secure a very comfortable standard of living. In 1532 he moved into one of the new houses on the western side of Piazza San Marco, next to the church of San Geminiano, a building that no longer exists today, for which he paid an annual rent of over twenty-five ducats. He also took full advantage of the fact that the city was the center of the European printing industry in the sixteenth century. At a time when some physicians were still reluctant to make use of the possibilities offered by the printing press, he grasped the opportunity the medium offered to further his career. He wrote short scientific texts and published them, at first in Latin and then more and more frequently in the vernacular, dealing with highly topical themes and exploring subjects that were to become increasingly popular. The only true limitation of his output was pointed out as early as the eighteenth century by Girolamo Tiraboschi, who, while recognizing Tommaso's "skill in treatment" as a doctor, criticized his "cumbersome and obscure" style of writing.[6] However, if we overlook this objective flaw, his works allow us to glimpse the full extent of the vitality of medical culture in sixteenth-century Venice.

His *Mali Galeci sanandi: vini ligni, & aquae, unctionis, ceroti, suffumigii, praecipitati, ac reliquorum modi omnes* was printed between 1537 and 1538, and it was extremely topical. The text focused on syphilis, a real scourge in Europe at the time, and it discussed its origins and looked at possible treatments, illustrating the preparation of formulas for syrups, pills, and poultices, some of which Rangone had concocted himself. This short document, which was published only in Latin because it was aimed at an educated readership, reveals Tommaso's relative modernity as a physician who was interested in the unfamiliar plant species that were arriving from the New World, and who was ready to make use of their healing powers. Tommaso devoted three enthusiastic chapters to *lignum vitae* (guaiacum), introduced to Europe by the Spanish in the first decade of the sixteenth century, and in subsequent editions he dedicated more and more space to the properties of exotic plants. The Biblioteca Nazionale Marciana in Venice still possesses a printed copy of the first edition of the *Mali Galeci*, studded with corrections and additions in Tommaso's own hand: a summary of the laboratory work of a Renaissance doctor who was aware of the development of scientific knowledge and at the same time the antigraph used for the typesetting of the second edition of 1545.[7] A third edition was brought out two years before his death (1575), with the number of pages increased by a third, many of them devoted to new botanical discoveries like cinchona, sarsaparilla, *caravalgio*, *huysan* root, and *mechiocan*, cited on the title page: an anthology of the novelties introduced as a result of what Tommaso repeatedly calls "Hispanorum diligentia [et] solertia" (Spanish diligence and ingenuity) and brought to Venice from the Americas by new trade routes. Another occasion to celebrate "Hispanorum diligentia [et] solertia", as well as "Lusitanorum navigatio" (Portuguese navigation), which had brought so many new medicinal plants to light, was provided by the publication of his *De vita hominis ultra CXX anno protrahenda* (1550). This was a thick quarto pamphlet of 120 sheets, reprinted in 1553 and 1560, and published once in the vernacular in 1556 "in a smaller volume for women," that is, in a reduced format (octavo) made up of only around eighty sheets.

His greatest success, however, was a slim work based on the model of the *regimen sanitatis* (rule of health), a genre whose manuscript tradition dated back to Classical Antiquity and which had flourished in the Middle Ages before taking on more popular forms with the invention of the printing press.[8] In 1565, 1570, and 1577 Tommaso published the *De vita Venetorum semper commoda Consilium*, both in Latin and in a vernacular translation, bringing out a total of eight editions (three of them in the vernacular 1577; the edition sometimes quoted as printed in 1558 is probably a bibliographic phantom). A handy octavo booklet of just sixteen sheets, it was a guide for the average Venetian to the so-called "six non-naturals", that is, the six external factors that influence health: air, food and drink, conditions of excretion and retention, exercise and rest, sleeping and waking, and the passions of the soul. The booklet examined the city's climate and its most common pathologies, providing advice on how to prevent them: it recommended frequent bathing and changes of clothing, carrying out all daytime and nighttime activities with the maximum restraint, avoiding intense passions, be they positive or negative, and applying moderation to the consumption of any kind of food. It was a modern text in its careful combination of the paradigm of prevention with the strictly therapeutic one of the medicinal secrets (or remedies) illustrated in other books: no medicine, argued Tommaso, could be effective if taken while leading a disorderly life.[9]

With an eye on Venetians' health and on the therapeutic innovations coming from the New World, Tommaso became much in demand as a doctor among both private individuals and local authorities. In 1534 he acted as medical officer to the Capitano Generale da Mar (admiral) Vincenzo Cappello and the following year he was asked by the health officials known as the Provveditori alla Sanità to write a report on how to clean the city's air.[10] In 1538 he was the medical officer for the Venetian fleet engaged in battle against the Turks. For the most part, however, Rangone consolidated his status as physician of the Venetians in the 1540s, with a clientele that included illustrious names such as the acclaimed architect Jacopo Sansovino, the sculptor Alessandro Vittoria (one of the executors of Tommaso's will), the troubled lawyer Mario d'Armano, nephew of painter Lorenzo Lotto, and many others.

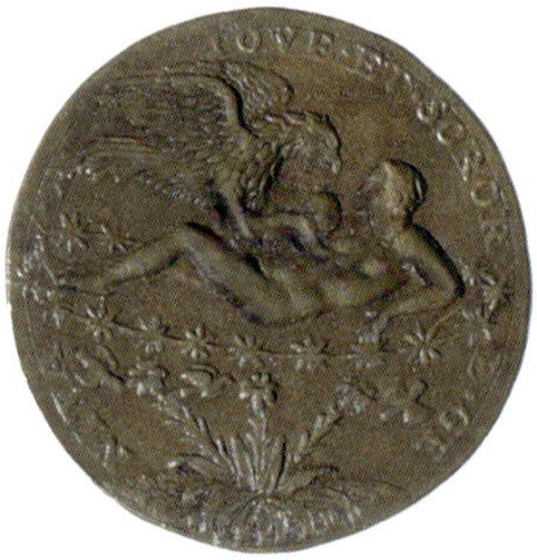

CAT. 71

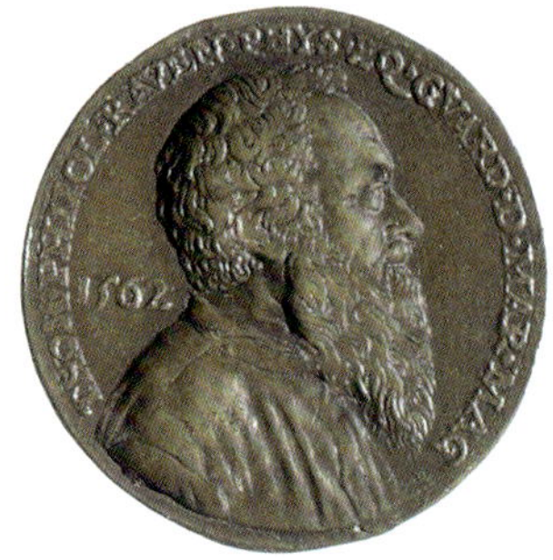

CAT. 72

CAT. 71, 72
MATTEO PAGANO (attrib.), *magnum* medal depicting *The Origin of the Milky Way* (verso) and with a *Portrait of Tommaso Giannotti Rangone* (recto), c. 1562

CAT 9.
DOMENICO TINTORETTO, *The Origin of the Milky Way* (from original by Jacopo Tintoretto, c. 1578–80), beginning of the seventeenth century

PALAZZO RAVENNA, THE MEDALS, AFFILIATIONS, AND COMMISSIONS OF ARTWORKS

Having made himself known through his "skill in treatment" and his books, from the early 1550s through to the 1560s, Tommaso carried out a series of initiatives that were both charitable and self-aggrandizing. Mindful of his own modest beginnings, in October 1552 he founded, in Padua's Palazzo Gritti, a building he had acquired, a college for thirty-two deserving students with limited means, to be recommended by Venetian parish priests. The same year, he struck the first of eight commemorative medals that he defined by their dimensions, *minimum*, *minus*, *medium*, *magnum*, and *maximum*. Some of these medals portrayed him in profile, while others illustrated myths or bore parenthetical or celebratory inscriptions. Five of them were the work of Alessandro Vittoria, one of Martino da Bergamo, and two of Matteo Pagano, an engraver and printer who had published the 1545 edition of the *Mali Galeci sanandi*. The production of medals was flourishing in Venice at the time, and Tommaso took advantage of its promotional potential, utilizing his medals — like his books — as visiting cards made of bronze, silver, and gold. At the time of their entry into Palazzo Ravenna, for example, members of the college received a *maximum* medal with his profile on one side and, on the other, a woman (representing Virtue) crowning an ox (Hard Work) in the presence of God, with the motto *Virtute parta Deo et labore* (Virtue Gained Through God and Works), executed with Alessandro Vittoria's typical stylistic concision.[11] When, in 1564, he became a member of the Venice College of Physicians, and one dispensed from payment of the *benintrada* (entrance fee) because he was at the peak of his career, Tommaso "gave [...] all the members of the College a silver medal with his likeness, and the College a book he had written *de proroganda vita usque ad annum 120*."[12]

Preceded to all intents and purposes by his own fame, Tommaso naturally found his way into the social fabric of the Venetian Republic. In 1559, he was admitted as a nobleman to the Scuola Grande di San Marco, of which he became Guardian Grande in 1562, and again in 1568, a privilege reserved for

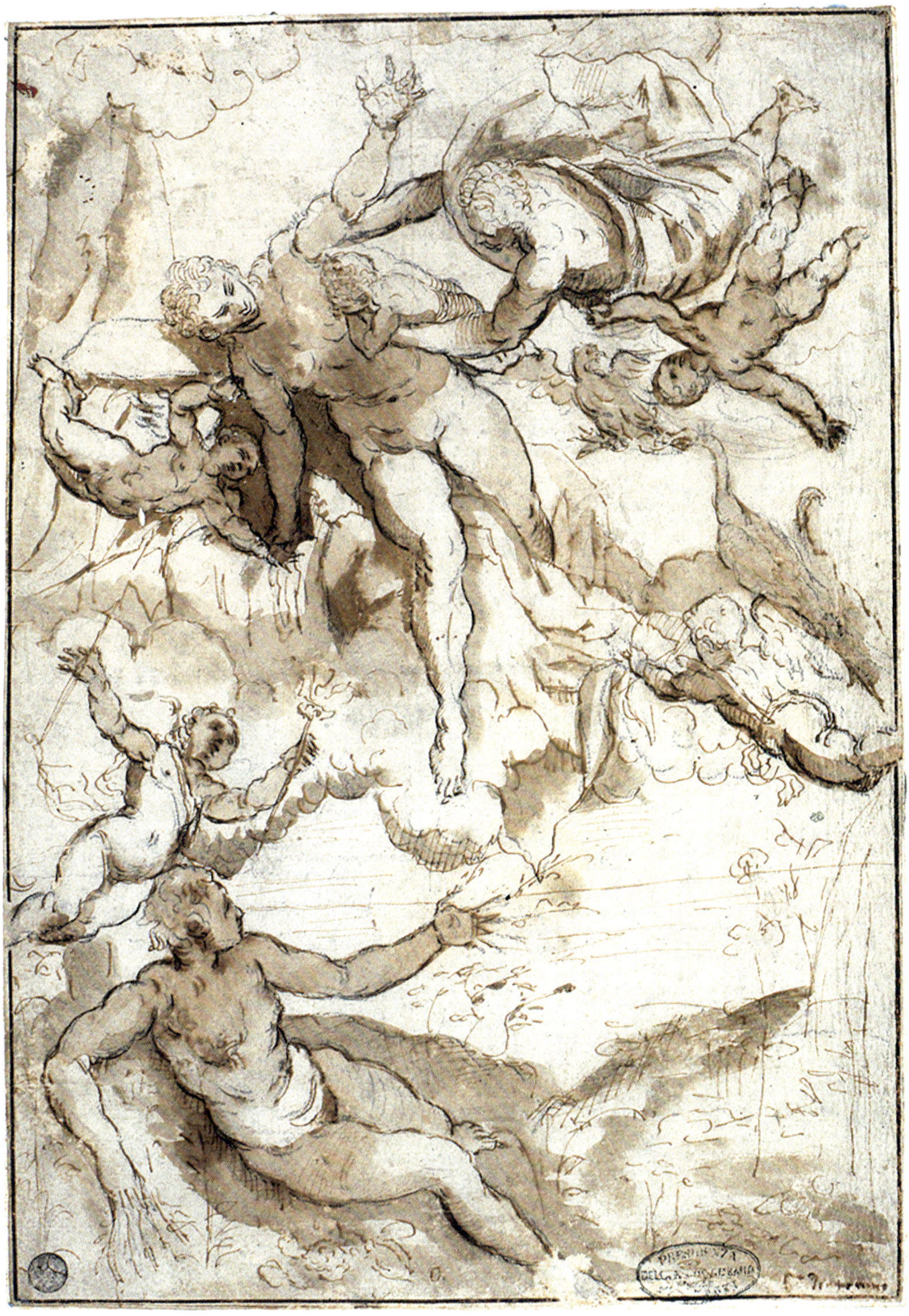

CAT. 9

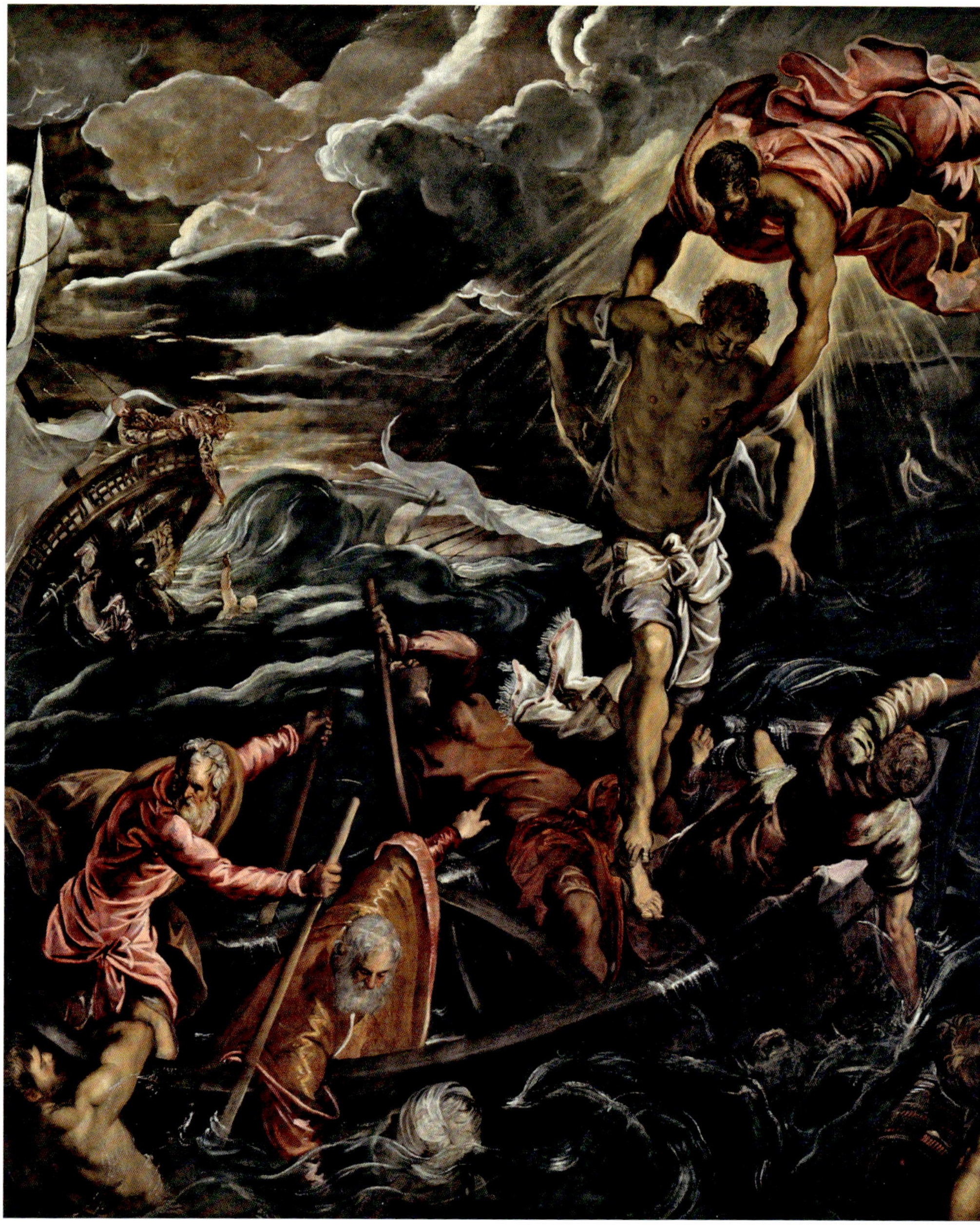

FIG. 6
JACOPO TINTORETTO,
Saint Mark Rescuing a Saracen from Shipwreck, c. 1564.
Venice, Gallerie dell'Accademia

native-born citizens of Venice or those who had belonged to the confraternity for at least twenty years, but which was barred to Venetian patricians.[13] He was also Guardian Grande of the Scuola di San Teodoro (1563), and procurator of a number of parish churches: San Geminiano, San Zulian, San Giovanni in Bragora, San Sepolcro, Santi Giovanni e Paolo, and Santa Maria dei Frari. The Venetian authorities only hindered his more self-aggrandizing initiatives, as they had been traditionally condemned in the oligarchic republic: in 1552 the Senate rejected Rangone's plan for a design for the façade of San Geminiano that had already been accepted by the parish church and commissioned from Sansovino, and ten years later the Scuola Grande di San Marco turned down the commission of a statue for its façade. Sometimes, fate got in the way. This was the case with the accord of April 1569, when Rangone was prior. In this year, the plan to build a new seat for the College of Physicians next to the church of San Geminiano, an extremely central location and one that was practically adjacent to his own home, fell through.[14]

Tommaso commissioned more and more works of art, and they were intertwined with one another, linked by frequent symbolic echoes. The year 1562 was a crucial one: Tommaso set up an annual grant of twenty ducats to provide dowries for poor girls on the feast day of Saint Geminianus; he was bestowed the title of Knight of Saint Mark by the doge; and he was appointed Guardian Grande of the Scuola di San Marco. To celebrate these honors he had Matteo Pagano strike a *magnum* medal (cat. 71–72) with a bust of him draped in a toga and crowned with his old and new titles on the recto, and a myth he was particularly fond of on the verso.[15] This device showed Jupiter in the form of an eagle holding the newborn Hercules to Juno's breast so he can suck the milk of immortality, while a few drops are scattered into the sky, giving rise to the Milky Way, and others, falling to earth, sprout as three lilies alternating with three birds. There are many correspondences with each other and with the divine: the Earth and living creatures (microcosm) are made of the same substance as the stars (macrocosm); the physician investigates both (flora in particular) to prolong the taste of immortality that the divine has allowed humanity. In addition, the three lilies and three birds were also elements of the coat of arms to which Tommaso had become entitled when he had assumed the title and surname of Count Rangone. It was a highly self-referential myth that symbolized his studies and his book on medicine, inspired by a Byzantine book on agriculture, the *Geoponica*, published in Venice a total of five times between 1538–54, in Italian and Latin. In chapter twenty, dedicated to the "History of the Lily," there is a precise description of the scene represented on the back of the medal. Also probably suggested, if not commissioned by Tommaso, was a painting by Jacopo Tintoretto that reworked the allegory of the medal cast by Pagano, *The Origin of the Milky Way* (c. 1575), only the upper two thirds of which have survived, and is now in London's National Gallery.[16] In the painting, the

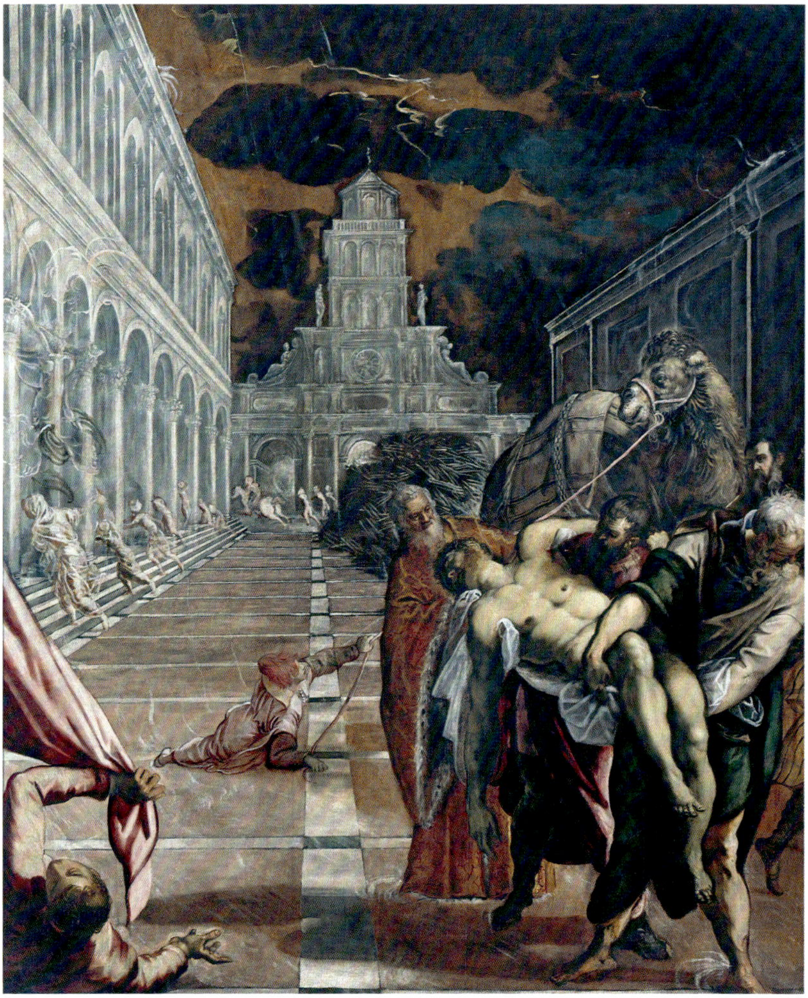

FIG. 7

medal's lilies were transformed into a female figure with fingers in the form of flowered branches (*Flora*), now visible only in a late seventeenth-century copy and in two drawings in watercolor and bister, one of which is in the Gallerie dell'Accademia in Venice (cat. 9).

Also in 1562, Rangone commissioned three large canvases from Tintoretto for the Sala Capitolare (Chapter Hall) of the Scuola Grande di San Marco: *Miracles of Saint Mark* (fig. 3), the *Rescue of the Body of Saint Mark* (fig. 7), and *Saint Mark Rescuing a Saracen from Shipwreck* (fig. 6). Tommaso makes an appearance in each scene, dressed in a patrician toga or in a glittering ducal robe. In 1573, irritated by the client's self-promotion, the brothers had the canvases taken down and returned to Tintoretto's studio so that he could finish them "perfectly by removing the figure of the Ravennate," but in the

FIG. 7
JACOPO TINTORETTO, *The Rescue of the Body of Saint Mark*, c. 1564. Venice, Gallerie dell'Accademia

end they were put back in place without alterations.[17] The ties between the forty-year-old Tintoretto and the physician in his sixties must have been strong. They certainly shared an aggressive style: Jacopo in the art market, which he liked to manipulate by offering pictures of large size painted in rapid and vigorous brushstrokes at knockdown prices or even by anticipating commissions; Rangone in the stubbornness with which he insinuated his own image into sacred and profane spaces.[18]

Tommaso's artistic projects always involved prominent figures that were turned into emblems of his personal mythical and allegorical constructions. To make up for the 1552 rejection of Tommaso's plans for San Geminiano's façade, Vittoria made a bronze bust for him that was located under the porch near the sacristy, and, in 1570, the sculptor also produced a statue of Saint Thomas — a metonym for himself — for the portal of the monastery of San Sepolcro. Vittoria produced the only monument to Tommaso that is still in place in the city: the bronze statue of his seated figure in the central lunette of the façade of San Zulian, built to Sansovino's design. Its celebration of Rangone's personal mythography is something that scholars are still interpreting in sophisticated ways today (fig. 8).[19] San Zulian's façade includes three inscriptions, in Latin, Greek, and Hebrew, which express Tommaso's trilingual aspirations and also describe the actions for which he wished to be remembered: in Greek, he told of the prestige he had imparted to the universities of Bologna, Padua, and Rome with his teaching; in Latin, he recalled how in San Zulian he had erected, with the money earned from his work, a temple to devotion, after having built one in Padua to excellence (Palazzo Ravenna), the latter a monument to the spirit and the former to the body as well; finally, in Hebrew, he spoke of himself as the author of many books and a doctor able to extend a patient's life.[20] At the sides of the bronze statue, bas-reliefs of the celestial (macrocosm) and terrestrial (microcosm) globe, above which extends the physician's arm with two shoots of plants from the New World, identifiable as guaiacum and sarsaparilla. All around are set bas-reliefs of open and closed books, laid flat and placed on a lectern, offering a summary of the sixteenth-century doctor's universe.

EPILOGUE: EIGHT OPEN BOOKS

For years Tommaso had been thinking about his last will and testament, although he did not have it definitively drawn up until a few days before his death, on September 10, 1577. The long will, originally compiled in triplicate, consisted largely of detailed instructions for the funeral procession, which had to pass through over a hundred places around the city, including the three most meaningful places of his life in Venice: San Geminiano, Santi Giovanni e Paolo, and San Zulian. Tommaso had also planned the display of about 260 books, his medals, portraits, drawings, astronomical instruments, and plans of the renovations he had funded. One of the will's more generous provisions

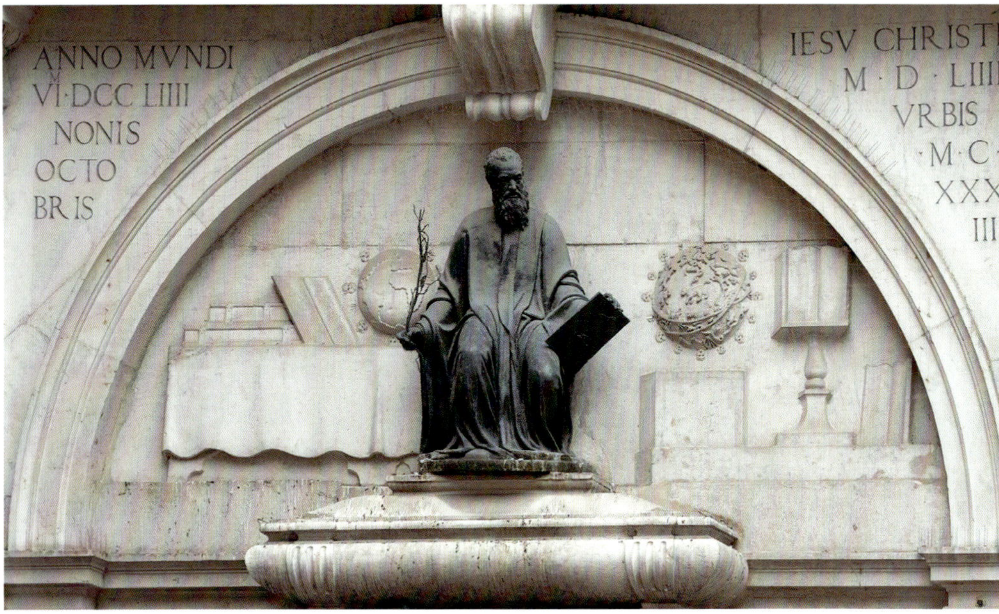

FIG. 8

was the donation of his magnificent personal library to the city for public use, with the acquisition of suitable premises in the central area of the Mercerie. Unfortunately, however, this plan was never realized: the books were transferred at first to the Capuchin library at Il Redentore, and then dispersed in 1810 following the Napoleonic suppressions. However, a partial inventory of that library (1561) has survived, along with a few copies of its books, still recognizable by their elegant, somber customized morocco binding, with linear gold tooling and the words *THOMAS* and *RAVENAS* in gold letters on the boards, sometimes accompanied by his coat of arms and other times by an ornament (cat. 36).

The procession certainly followed the planned route, though perhaps with less pomp than Tommaso would have liked, as the city had only recently emerged from an outbreak of the plague (1575–76). This is how the event was recorded by the College of Physicians on September 13, 1577:

> Funeral of Tomaso Philologist from Ravenna famous doctor and d. at the age of 94 [actually 84] *vivens semper sine ulla corporis molestia* having survived the danger of contagion, and ordered among other things that three funeral orations be given, one in San Giminian his parish church and made by a Rev. priest, one in San Gio. Polo and made by Belisario Gadaldin, one in San Giulian where his body is laid.[21]

While not as many as he would have desired, he was almost certainly accompanied on his last journey by the set of eight volumes that he wanted to be placed open around his coffin.

FIG. 8
ALESSANDRO VITTORIA, *Portrait of Tommaso Giannotti Rangone*, c. 1556–57. Venice, façade of the church of San Zulian

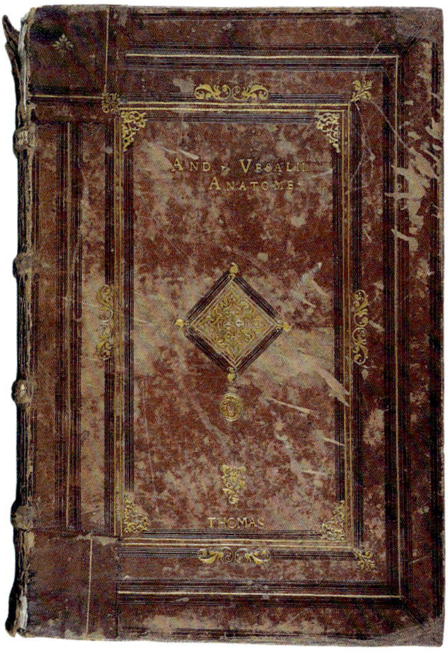

CAT. 36

First, behind his head, he wanted the history of the city of his birth, Ravenna, open to a precise page. It was probably a magnificent illustrated manuscript of large format, like the other volumes.[22]

Second, Rangone selected Vesalius's *Fabrica* and *Epitome*, which doubtlessly was the majestic printed volume now held in the Biblioteca Marciana, with Tommaso's original binding, and described in the inventory of his library as "Vesalii Anatome seu Humani corporis fabrica Epithome, Basilee impressi 1543 folio reali maximo corio rubro auro decorata ac litteris."[23] Bound together, the book comprises Andreas Vesalius's masterpiece, *De humani corporis fabrica libri septem* (Basel 1543), and his *De humani corporis fabrica librorum Epitome*, with the same colophon, whose twelve foldout plates presented the most up-to-date anatomical knowledge of the day. It is even possible for us to identify at precisely which plates it was kept open on the day of the funeral at Tommaso's behest, since they are indicated in the will as the "tertia et secunda humana figura masculos [*sic*] demonstrante bini completa" (cat. 36).

The next three volumes he wanted displayed around him were part of an unpublished work by Giannotti on the natural kingdoms, also opened at precise illustrations: the volume on quadrupeds shows two fantastical animals (the asymmetrical *daru* or *dahu*, whose legs were believed to be shorter on one side than on the other, and the *hircocervus*, believed to be half-goat and half-stag); the one on birds must have shown a bird of paradise from New Guinea, as well as a crow and a European roller; the one on sea life showed the sea cucumber, a starfish-like echinoderm, and the *sea monk*, a fanciful interpretation of a giant squid.

CAT. 36
ANDREAS VESALIUS,
Andreae Vesalii Bruxellensis, ... De humani corporis fabrica...,
Basel, 1543

TERTIA MVSCVLOS OSTENDENTIVM FIGVRA, PRIMAM ET SECVNDAM

QVITVR, MVSCVLOS ILLIS QVOS IPSAE SINISTRIS LATERIBVS REFEREBANT PROX

succumbentes, dextro latere in anteriori facie proponens, dein sinistro atere illos referens qui dextri lateris subsunt musculis ter linguæ & laryngis musculos, & cartilagines hic humi repositas. Cerebri uerò partium hic nihil propter capitis in post reflexum occurrit.

DEXTRI LATERIS CHARACterum Index.

- A Palatum adhuc obductum tunica.
- B Gargeon
- C Tert maxillam mouentium. est enim hic maxille ad summum mentum dissecta, & utrinque ad latera ducta.
- D Dextra pars inferioris maxillæ.
- E,F Duo quarti maxillam mouentium musculi uentres. G Neruea sedes inter eos uentres consistens.
- H Laryngis operculum.
- I Altera tonsilla.
- K Lingua.
- L Quintus linguæ musculus.
- N,N Dexter υ referens os ad latera trahentiū.
- O Dexter duorum à pectoris osse in scuti imaginem exprimentem laryngis cartilaginem insertorum.
- P Asperæ arteriæ caudex.
- Q Dexter primi paris dorsum agentium.
- R Dexter secundi paris dorsum agentium.
- S Portio secundi paris caput mouentium.
- T Portio tertij scapulam mouentium.
- V Series neruorum axillam petentium.
- X Pectoris os.
- Y,Y Costarum ossa.
- g,g Costarum cartilagines.
- h,h Intercostalium exteriorum series in ossium interuallis.
- i,i Intercostalium exteriorum series in cartilaginum interuallis.
- k,k Secundus thoracem mouentium.
- l Cartilaginis in quam pectoris os exacuitur sedes.
- m Rectus abdominis musculus a,b,c,d circunscriptus.
- n Vmbilici relicta portio.
- o Transuersi abdominis musculi magna portio.
- p Seminalia uasa hic sunt præsecta.
- q Penis corporum hic conspicitur substantia.
- r Meatus urinæ ac semini communis.
- ſ Septimus brachium mouentium.
- t Quintus brachium mouentium.
- u Interior scapulæ processus.
- x Brachij os.
- y Tertius brachium mouentium.
- α Quarti brachium mouentium insertionis portio.
- β Primus cubitum extendentium.
- γ Posterior cubitum flectentium.
- δ Primus radium in pronum agentium.
- ε Insertio anterioris cubitum extendentium.
- ζ Primus radium in supinum ducentium.
- η Secundus digitos mouentium, a,b,c circunscriptus.
- θ Tertius digitos manus mouentiū, cuius tendo a indicatur.
- ι Minor primorum duorum pollicis os flectentium.
- λ,μ,ν,ξ Quatuor musculi quatuor digitos pollici adducentes.
- ο Exterior duorum primum parui digiti os flectentium.
- π Ilium ossis spina hic excarnis modò uisitur.
- ρ Portio tertij femur mouentium.
- σ Septimi femur mouentium portio.
- τ Sexti femur mouentium portio.
- υ Octauus femur mouentium.
- φ Quinti femur mouentium portio.
- χ Maior exterior'ue femoris processus.
- ψ Septimus tibiam mouentium, a,b,c circunscriptus.
- ω Octauus tibiam mouentiū, d,e,f etiam insignitus, magnaq; adhuc portione sub septimo latitans.
- Γ Tendo noni tibiam mouentium.
- Δ,Δ Tibiæ ossis excarnis pars.
- Θ Decimusquintus digitos pedis mouentium.
- Λ Portio septimi pedem mouentium.
- Ξ Decimussextus digitos mouentium.
- Γ Tendo tertij pedem mouentium.
- Σ,Σ Quartus pedem mouentium.
- Υ Hic tendo primi & secundi pedem mouentium quarto con nascitur unitur q; musculo, estq; hic præsectus.
- Ω Portio secundi pedis digitos mouentium.
- ı,ı Portiones sunt transuersorum harū sedium ligamentorū.

SINISTRI LATERIS CHARACterum Index.

- A Propago minoris radicis tertij paris neruorum cerebri, quæ cuti frontis offertur.
- B Dictæ radicis propago, nariū amplitudinē petens.
- C Propago dictæ radicis, superiorē accedens maxillā.
- D Quarti paris neruorū cerebri series in palati tunicā.
- E Maioris tertij paris radicis propago, instar capreoli inuoluta.
- F Dictæ radicis portio linguam petens.

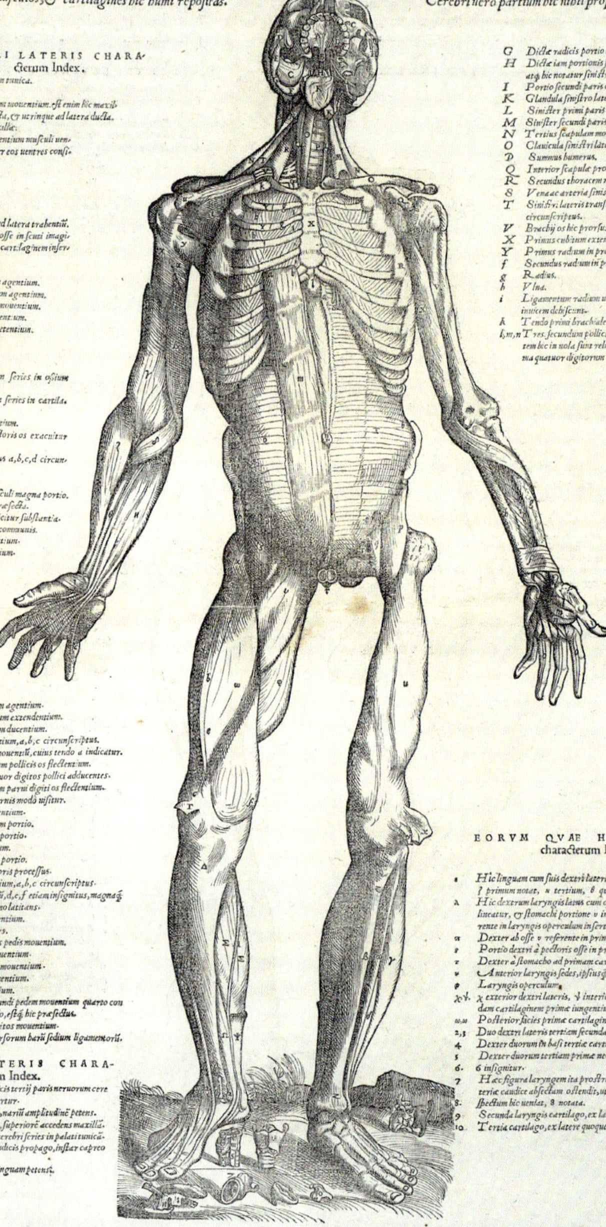

- G Dictæ radicis portio inferiori maxillæ d strib
- H Dictæ iam portionis soboles inferiori labro dep atq; hic notatur sinistra inferioris maxillæ pars.
- I Portio secundi paris caput mouentium.
- K Glandula sinistro lateri laryngis subnata.
- L Sinister primi paris caput mouentium.
- M Sinister secundi paris caput mouentium.
- N Tertius scapulam mouentium.
- O Clauicula sinistri lateris.
- P Summus humerus.
- Q Interior scapulæ processus.
- R Secundus thoracem mouentium.
- S Vena ac arteria sinistro pectoris ossi exporre
- T Sinistri lateris transuersus abdominis musculus circunscriptus.
- V Brachij os hic prorsus nudum conspicitur.
- X Primus cubitum extendentium.
- Y Primus radium in pronum ducentium.
- f Secundus radium in pronum agentium.
- g Radius.
- h Vlna.
- i Ligamentum radium ulnæ inibi committens, ubi invicem dehiscunt.
- k Tendo primi brachiale mouentium.
- l,m,n Tres secundum pollicis internodium flectentes tem hic in uola sunt reliqui, octo illi censentur, q ma quatuor digitorum ossa flectuntur.
- o,o Transuersa dig gamenta indican bus primi & secu tos mouentium te ducebantur.
- p Septimi femur m portio.
- q Sexti femur mou portio.
- r,r Pubis os sinistrum
- ſ Nonus femur m tium.
- t Exterior maior' ris processus.
- u Octauus tibiam tium, qui uniuersu si femoris os pr ambit.
- x Portio tendinis femur mouentium
- y Tendo noni tibi uentium.
- Tibiæ os.
- α Fibula.
- β Ligamentum m neum fibulam tibi gans.
- γ Septimus pedem tium.
- δ Octauus pedem tium. Superior pedis sedes omnin excarnis est, ipsiu ligamētis adhuc conspiciuntur.
- Posterior tibiæ dextro cruri resp

EORVM QVAE HVMI IACN characterum Index.

- ι Hic linguam cum suis dextri lateris musculis delineauimus, ζ primum notat, κ tertium, θ quintum, ι septimum, κ
- λ Hic dextrum laryngis latus cum osse υ referente, & μ no lineatur, & stomachi portione υ indicata. ξ musculi ab osse rente in laryngis operculum inserti.
- α Dexter ab osse υ referente in primam cartilaginem insertor
- ρ Portio dextri à pectoris osse in primam cartilaginem inse
- τ Dexter à stomacho ad primam cartilaginem pertinentium.
- υ Anterior laryngis sedes, ipsiusq; primæ cartilaginis imag
- φ Laryngis operculum.
- χ ψ. χ exterior dextri lateris, ψ interior sinistri lateris quatuor dam cartilaginem primæ iungentium.
- ω,ω Posterior facies primæ cartilaginis.
- 2,3 Duo dextri lateris tertiam secundæ iungentium.
- 4 Dexter duorum in basi tertiæ cartilaginis positorum.
- 5 Dexter duorum tertiam primæ nectentium · sinistri autem
- 6. 6 insignitur.
- 7 Hæc figura laryngem ita prostratam, atque à reliquo asp teriæ caudice abscectam ostendit, ut ipsius rimula seu lingula
- 8. spectum hic ueniat, 8 notata.
- 9 Secunda laryngis cartilago, ex latere dextro expressa.
- 10 Tertia cartilago, ex latere quoque dextro delineata.

SECV

CAT. 36

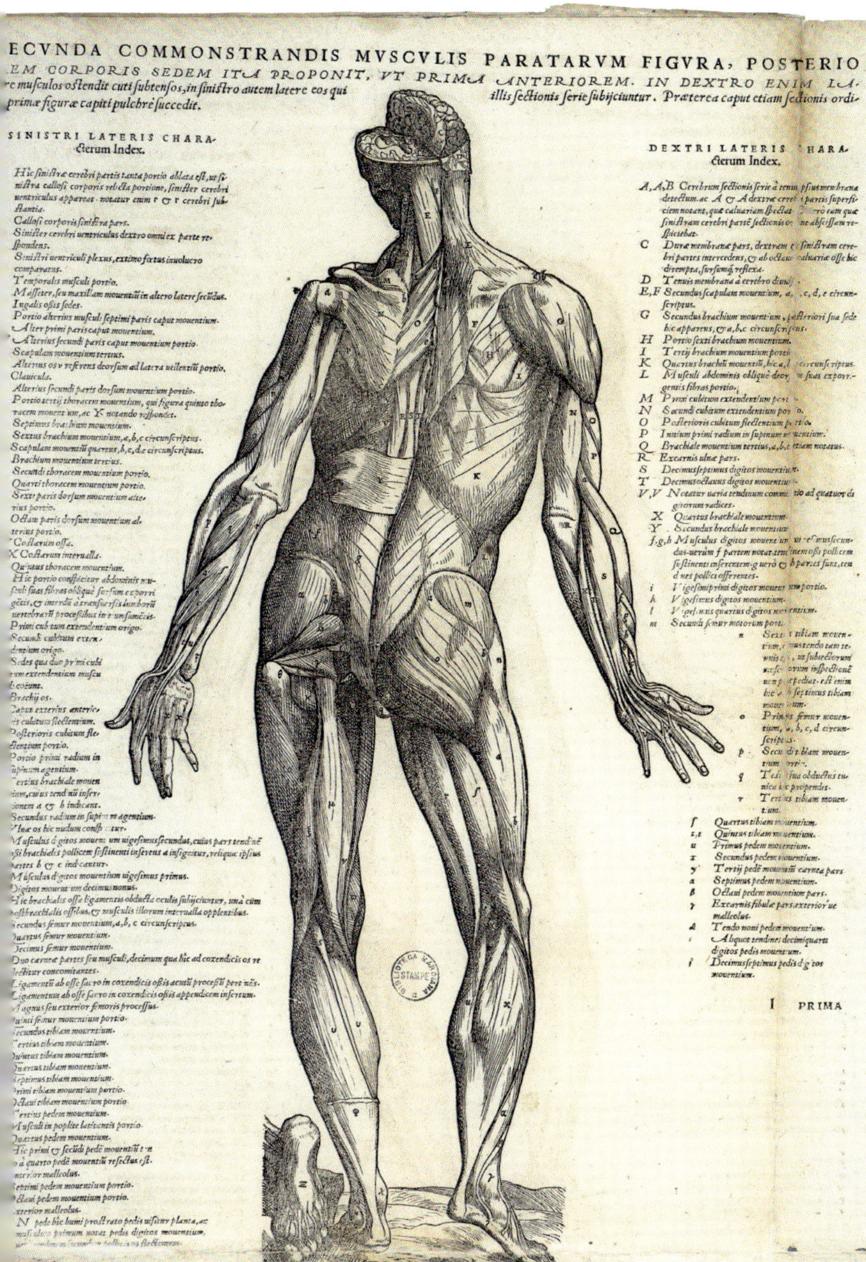
ECVNDA COMMONSTRANDIS MVSCVLIS PARATARVM FIGVRA, POSTERIO
EM CORPORIS SEDEM ITA PROPONIT, VT PRIMA ANTERIOREM. IN DEXTRO ENIM LA-
re musculos ostendit cuti subtensos, in sinistro autem latere eos qui illis sectionis serie subijciuntur. Praeterea caput etiam sectionis ordi-
primae figurae capiti pulchrè succedit.
SINISTRI LATERIS CHARActerum Index.
DEXTRI LATERIS CHARActerum Index.
I PRIMA

For the sixth volume, devoted to simple plants used for their medicinal properties, Tommaso chose the *Commentarii in sex libros Pedacii Dioscoridis Anazarbei de Medica Materia* by Pietro Andrea Mattioli, open at the colored woodcuts of the *Peonia mascula et foemina* on pages 914–15. The edition referred to is the Venetian Folio One printed by Vincenzo Valgrisi in 1565, the only one in which the illustrations are on those pages.

Tommaso's seventh choice belonged to the genre of Catholic devotion: a Roman Missal open at the engraving of *Christ Crucified* ("Missali a sole majori cartis 130 Jesus Christus cruci affixus") that coincides with the rare "Missale a sole reali folio Venetiis, a Juntis 1557" in his library: an illustrated folio volume with a splendid woodcut of *Christ Crucified* on sheet 130v.

To crown this translation of the human, animal, and vegetable microcosm into book form, Tommaso selected the "Ptolommei Cosmographia respiciens mapamundo," that is, the woodcut world map of the Strasbourg edition of 1525, the *Geographicae enarrationis libri octo*, of which he possessed a copy in his library: "Cosmographia vulgo Ptolomei Geographia impressa 1525 folio reali, corio vario aureo filo ac litteris cum annotationibus Montis Regii cum tabulis Terrae nove et modernis." Rangone's interest in geography was deep and constant, as the Veronese engraver Paolo Forlani declared when dedicating the plate of Africa to him on May 9, 1562.[24]

Altogether, these eight volumes are the fruit of the bibliographical choices of a Renaissance physician who tried to keep as up-to-date as possible; they include the most innovative printed texts and personal compilations (the ones on the animal kingdoms), where exhaustive printed editions were still lacking. Vesalius's *Fabrica* and *Epitome* represented a high point in anatomical studies owing to the critical attitude they took to ward the authorities of classical anatomy, who were corrected and amended in light of what had been learned from the practice of dissection — a critical revision that some within academic circles found hard to accept. The *Commentarii a Dioscoride* of the Sienese doctor Mattioli were, after Vesalius, the most significant example of medico-scientific publishing in the sixteenth century, with fundamental effects on the field of pharmacology. Most notably, Mattioli correctly identified the medicinal plants described, in the first century AD, by Dioscorides, whose writings had been corrupted in the process of copying the manuscripts; and, in each edition, Mattioli added new plants and descriptions, tripling the number of simple plants and thus the stock of medicinal herbs that European apothecaries could use with confidence. Finally, Ptolemy's *Geographia* (first-second centuries AD), but with the corrections made by Regiomontanus, represented an important step toward modern geography, with maps of new and modern lands, as Tommaso explained in the inventory of his library. These new lands were also the source of innovation in treatments offered by medicine in his century.

previous pages
CAT. 36
ANDREAS VESALIUS, *Andreae Vesalii Bruxellensis, ... De humani corporis fabrica librorum Epitome*, Basel, 1543

NOTES

1 E. Weddigen, "Thomas Philologus Ravennas. Gelehrter, Wohltäter und Mäzen," in *Saggi e memorie di storia dell'arte*, 9 (1974), 7–76, and F. Bacchelli, entry, *Dizionario Biografico degli Italiani* (Rome: Istituto della Enciclopedia Italiana, 2000), Vol. 54; S. Herrmann, *Tomaso Rangone: Arzt, Astrologe und Mäzen im Italien der Renaissance* (Göttingen: Vandenhoeck & Ruprecht, 2016).

2 *Permissu inuictissimi artistarum et medicorum studii Bononiensis... Stephani Strutii Parmensis rectoris clarissimi sub... Pamphilo Monte... Thomas philologus Ianothus Rhauennas de conclusionibus his dissertabit*, Archivio di Stato di Bologna, CNCE 69133, s.is a.e. e.e. o.i. (C) 1513 (Q) (EDIT16: http://edit16.iccu.sbn.it/web__iccu/imain.htm).

3 Twenty-five prognostications that he published in Latin and Italian between 1513 and 1525 have survived (see EDIT16).

4 "Lettera di Tommaso a Federico duca di Mantova e marchese di Monferrato, Venezia 8 Febbraio 1538," *Il bibliofilo*, 8 (1887), 78.

5 E. Garin, *Lo zodiaco della vita: la polemica sull'astrologia dal Trecento al Cinquecento* (Rome and Bari: Laterza, 2007).

6 G. Tiraboschi, *Storia della letteratura italiana* (Rome: Luigi Perego Salvioni, 1784), Vol. 7.2, 60.

7 Biblioteca Nazionale Marciana (henceforth BNM), Ms. Lat. VII 37(=3601).

8 K. Albala, *Eating Right in the Renaissance* (Berkeley and Los Angeles: University of California Press, 2002).

9 S. Cavallo and T. Storey, *Healthy Living in Late Renaissance Italy* (Oxford: Oxford University Press, 2013).

10 *Ad clarissimos salutis iustissimae urbis Venetiarum praesides... De repentini mortiferis, & ut ita dicam, miraculosis nostri temporis aegritudinibus* (Venice, 1535).

11 C. Crisafulli and L. Mezzaroba, "La Scuola medaglistica veneziana nel Rinascimento attraverso le collezioni del Museo Correr," *Bollettino dei Musei Civici Veneziani*, 4, *Le medaglie rinascimentali di Scuola veneziana nelle collezioni dei Musei civici veneziani* (2009), 7–67, no. 108.

12 BNM, Ms. It. VII 2342(=9695), c. 12v.

13 On this subject, see the essay by P. Benussi.

14 BNM, Ms. It. VII 2342(=9695), c. 14v.

15 Crisafulli and Mezzaroba 2009, no. 111.

16 N. Penny, "The Origin of the Milky Way," in *The Sixteenth Century Italian Paintings*, Vol. 2: *Venice 1540-1600* (London: National Gallery, 2008), 154–63.

17 See "Chronology."

18 T. Nichols, *Tintoretto. Tradition and Identity* (London: Reaktion Books, 1999), 137–43.

19 M. Morresi, *Jacopo Sansovino* (Electa: Milan 2000), 132–34, 262–64, 297–305; A. Gallo, "In forma di microcosmo. Tommaso Filologo e il portale della chiesa di San Zulian," in *Cose nuove e cose antiche. Scritti per monsignor Antonio Niero e don Bruno Bertoli*, ed. F. Cavazzana Romanelli, M. Leonardi, and S. Rossi Minutelli (Venice: Biblioteca Nazionale Marciana, 2006), 493–510.

20 N. Zorzi, "L'iscrizione trilingue di Tommaso Rangoni sulla facciata della chiesa di San Zulian a Venezia (1554)," *Quaderni per la storia dell'Università di Padova*, 45 (2012), 107–37.

21 BNM, Ms. It. VII 2342(=9695), c. 17r.

22 ASVe, *Notarile testamenti*, b. 421, no. 1172, c. 4v, for this and the subsequent quotations.

23 S. Minuzzi, "Il medico Tommaso Giannotti Rangone (1493–1577) nell'economia della cura ovvero un trionfo di libri, segreti e *regimen sanitatis*," *Medicina & Storia*, n.s., 1 (2013), 29–66, for precise references to the inventory (BNM, Ms. lat. XIV, 282(= 4298), cc. 84–125).

24 The British Library, London, Cartographic Items, Maps K. Top.117.1.

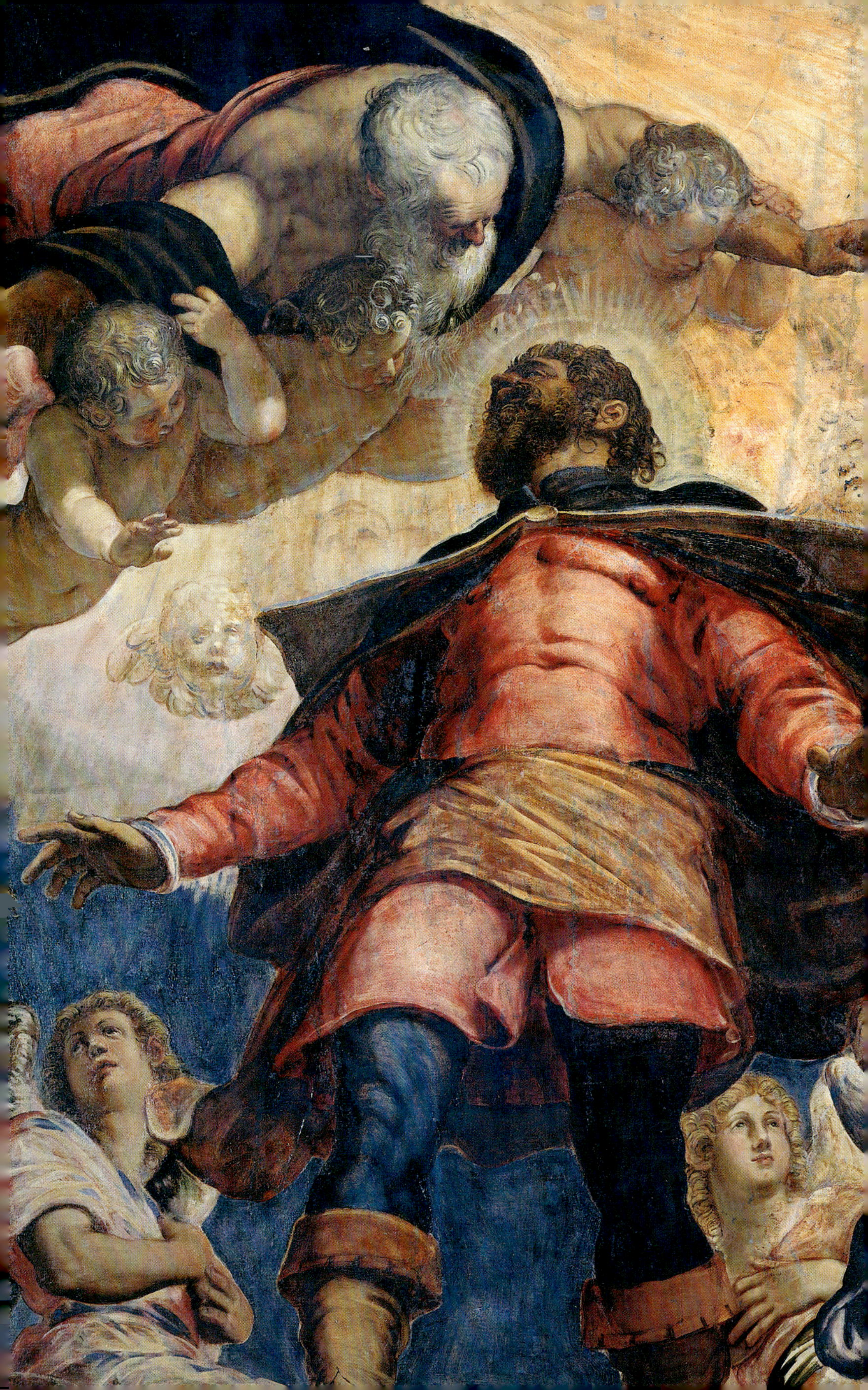

'WHEN GOD'S MAJESTY PUBLICLY SCOURGES A PEOPLE': COMBATING PLAGUE IN SIXTEENTH-CENTURY VENICE

Michelle Laughran

REFERENCES TO PLAGUE (*peste* in Italian) pervade the historical record, testimony to humanity's extreme vulnerability to disease for most of our history. Indeed, the word has at times been used so broadly that it merely signified an epidemic. Jacopo Tintoretto, for example, probably witnessed at least nine such massive ones over the course of his lifetime.[1] The word "plague," however, was applied most famously to the virulent Black Death, the pandemic that decimated the population of Europe, starting in 1347–48, and then returning at least once per generation over the course of the next four centuries.[2]

Venice had been one of the first cities to invoke a special governmental committee back in 1348 to combat that grave health emergency. During each subsequent wave of epidemic, the government would reconvene a similar committee. Fortunately for Tintoretto and his fellow Venetian citizens, this ad-hoc committee was elevated to the status of a permanently standing public health administration during the outbreak of 1486. These officials, called the Provveditori alla Sanità, expanded their jurisdiction over the course of the next century until it included urban sanitation, licensing medical practitioners, overseeing the quality of drinking water and foodstuffs for sale, and controlling the city's populations of sex workers and the impoverished. For potential health threats, this office (like other magistracies of the Venetian Republic) accepted anonymous denunciations slipped into so-called "lion's mouth" collection slots around the city (fig. 9) and was empowered to impose whatever corporal punishments against the condemned it deemed fit, including public shaming, whipping, or imprisonment for anyone who transgressed in matters of the Provveditori's extensive public health jurisdictions.

This era, however, did not view disease control in medical terms only. Collective spiritual actions like the ritual flagellation practiced by the Scuola Grande di San Marco had been employed ever since the Black Death in penitential attempts to secure God's mercy. In 1486, the same year the Provveditori were established, members of the Venetian confraternity of San Rocco likewise sought additional heavenly protections against plague by acquiring that saint's relics. With Roch's body then permanently residing in Venice, the plague saint not only enhanced the fortunes and prestige of his titular Scuola Grande but, importantly, he also served as a kind of holy prophylaxis for the city.

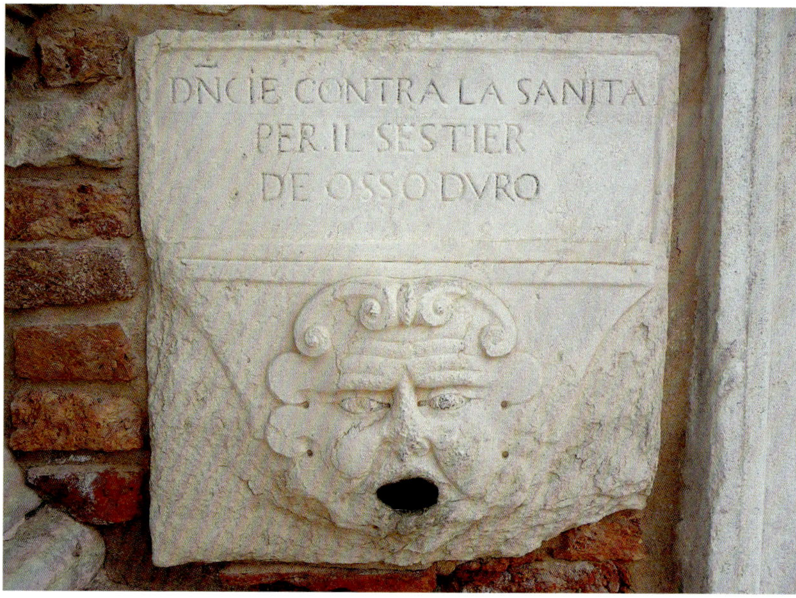
DÑCIE CONTRA LA SANITA
PER IL SESTIER
DE OSSO DVRO

FIG. 9

FIG. 9
Lion's mouth collection slot for anonymous denunciations of public health offenses to the Provveditori alla Sanità. Sestiere of Dorsoduro, Venice

Interestingly, the frequency of plague episodes does actually seem to have decreased from the fifteenth century onward, and both Saint Roch and the Provveditori were at the time credited with what seemed to be their successful interventions. In cases of outbreak, the Provveditori were charged with diagnosing the epidemic and executing the appropriate response. Most feared of all was the bubonic form of plague associated with the Black Death.[3] The characteristic "buboes" that gave the affliction its name were large swellings of the lymph nodes which were excruciatingly painful. To get a sense of these terrifying abscesses now, one need only glance at a Renaissance depiction of Saint Roch himself: a huge bubo on the inner thigh was the saint's most identifiable attribute, depicted beneath his clothes in Tintoretto's glorious *Apotheosis of Saint Roch* (fig. 10), and more graphically suppurating in the depictions from the previous century by his predecessors. When the disease finally overran the infected gland, afflicted individuals would suffer severe headaches, high fever, and carbuncles or petechial spotting on the skin, with death following within a matter of just a few days in an estimated 40–60% of cases.

When "true plague" was suspected in an epidemic, quarantine would be imposed. First utilized in the fourteenth century by the Venetian subject city of Dubrovnik (known in Italian as Ragusa), these measures would be adopted by the Republic, starting in 1423. Since Venice was uniquely able to take advantage of its many lagoon islands, by the sixteenth century the Provveditori alla Sanità were responsible for administering a network of

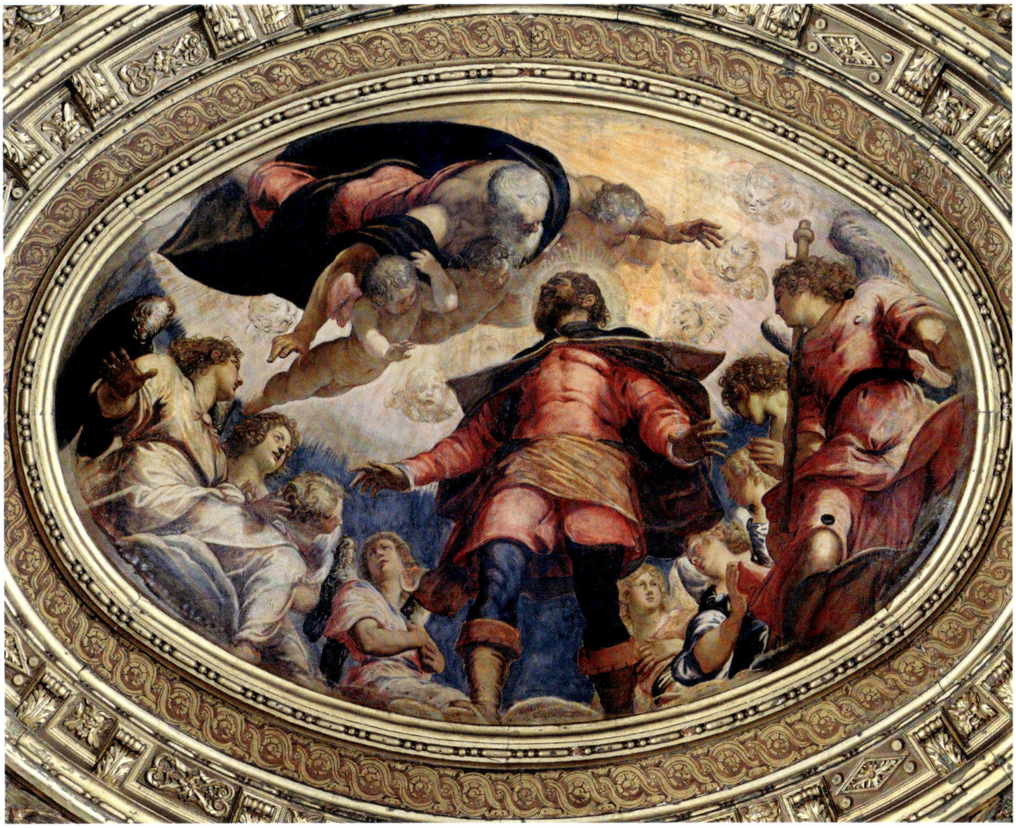

FIG. 10

graduated quarantines around the city aimed at reducing contact between potential disease carriers and the population at large as much as possible. These hapless persons were housed in segregated holding areas for around forty days or, in Italian, "una quarantina di giorni," thereby giving the influential public health procedure its name. And since this network included what seems to have been Europe's first permanent plague hospital on the nearby island of Santa Maria di Nazareth (next to the island of San Lazzaro), Venice would thus inspire the name for all such subsequent institutions: *lazzaretto* (fig. 11). During particularly large-scale epidemics, the Health Office could take Venetian quarantine even further by sealing off individual houses, whole city blocks, or even entire parishes, and when an outbreak was raging too quickly to be accommodated by the two permanent *lazzaretti*, other lagoon islands could be commandeered into the process as well.[4]

FIG. 10
JACOPO TINTORETTO, *Apotheosis of Saint Roch*, 1564. Venice, Scuola Grande di San Rocco

The Provveditori alla Sanità did not utilize hospitals only for the quarantine of those known to have been in proximity of infectious disease during a time of plague. In 1528, an epidemic hit the city at the same time that a famine was dramatically raising the prices of grain throughout

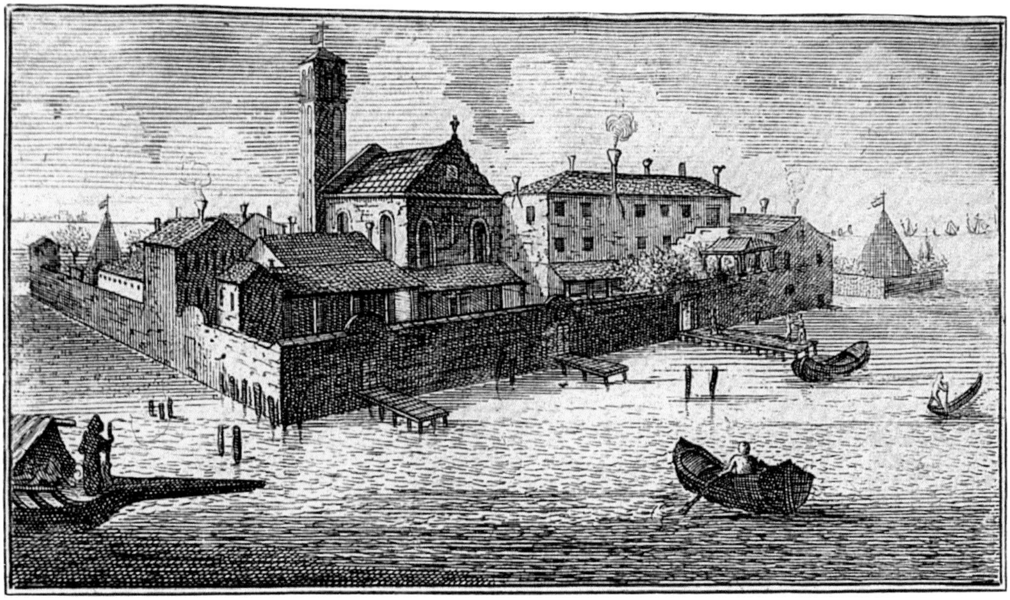

FIG. 11

the Veneto region. As the outbreak seemed to be disproportionately targeting the poor in the city — the ranks of whom were swelling daily with continued influx from the mainland — the Venetian Republic decreed that a hospital for the poor should be founded in an open field where a makeshift refugee camp had arisen near the Dominican friary of Santi Giovanni e Paolo. This hospital, formally named Santa Maria dei Derelitti and colloquially called the Ospedaletto (Little Hospital), would eventually host "many thousands of the wretched poor [including] the sick, the derelict [...] boys and girls, orphans, and others of every needy sort."[5] It formed the initial foundation of an area hospital network that would subsequently include the late sixteenth-century hospital of San Lazzaro dei Mendicanti, thereby laying the foundations for Venice's Ospedale Civile today.

Although medical experts may have frequently applauded efforts to hospitalize the poor and to quarantine the sick, they could be divided in their reasoning as to why such measures should be efficacious.[6] No fewer than 280 plague treatises had been written between the first outbreak of the Black Death in 1347–48 and 1500 and — counting just the Italian printing houses alone — the number of individual titles likely doubled over the course of the next century. As physicians and other authors grappled in text with explaining the affliction's terrifying and often unpredictable behavior, plague tracts seem to have become one of the earliest forms of popular literature in the West.[7]

FIG. 11
FRANCESCO ZUCCHI, *Isola del Lazaretto Vecchio* in *Teatro delle fabbriche più cospicue in prospettiva, sì pubbliche che private della città di Venezia*, published by Giambattista Albrizzi q. Girolamo, 1740. Venice, Biblioteca Nazionale Marciana

Among these, plague treatises informed by academic medicine were heavily influenced by the classical theories of Hippocrates and Galen and generally taught that diseases resulted from an imbalance of humors, the fluids considered the body's source of health and wellbeing. An epidemic in typical humoral logic was believed to have resulted from an area-wide contamination of the environment, which simultaneously destabilized many individuals' constitutions. Side-by-side with this Galenic conception of the plague, however, another theory suggested that it was spread through person-to-person contact. This latter theory was most fully articulated by Girolamo Fracastoro when, reflecting upon numerous virulent sicknesses like plague and, most notably, syphilis,[8] he sought to reconcile humoral explanations of the origins of diseases with what seemed to be infections via individuals and/or their possessions. "It is manifest that the seeds of contagion arise first in ourselves," he wrote in his 1546 publication *De Contagione*.[9] When such infectious "seeds" were spontaneously generated through the process of putrefaction, Fracastoro claimed they could be passed directly from person to person through touch, indirectly through the handling of shared objects, or potentially even at a distance by a mere glance when no direct or indirect contact had seemingly transpired.

Whether the epidemic was thought to have been generated by pestilential miasmas or by contagion, plague was nonetheless believed to act upon the infected human body like a poison. As a result, the preferred pharmaceutical remedy of the time was the famed poison antidote, *teriaca*. An estimated 600,000 pounds of this medicinal was produced annually by Venice's forty licensed apothecaries, and indeed its very name in English — Venetian treacle — was testament to the city's reputation for producing the finest.[10]

Similarly, the strange costume of the Venetian plague doctor (fig. 12) which appeared during the seventeenth century was designed to shield its wearer from head to toe regardless of whether disease was perpetuated by putrefying miasmas or by contagious "seeds." The peculiar beaklike mask would be stuffed with aromatic sachets which were thought to purify the infectious stench in the air, while its rose-colored lenses provided extra protection from the potentially contagious gaze of the sick.[11]

Eventually, hospitals, quarantines, and *cordons sanitaires* throughout Europe became so efficient at controlling the spread of diseases that their implementation may have contributed to the elimination of bubonic plague from mainland Europe after 1720. In the sixteenth century, however, cities were still reluctant to implement these measures, because of the severe disruptions they caused to trade between cities and to the social fabric within them. The wide-ranging disruptions generated by quarantine, coupled with contemporaries' varying conceptions of plague and its causes, meant that officials and physicians could at times be fiercely divided regarding the nature of a given outbreak and thus the best measures to combat it.

Notably, the catastrophic epidemic of 1575–77 was the occasion for just such a dramatic difference in opinion. In 1576, before the summer — peak time not only for shipping but also, potentially, for disease — the Venetian government had looked to medical professors from the nearby University of Padua to confirm whether the full quarantine protocols advocated by the city's Provveditori alla Sanità to limit the previous year's outbreak were truly necessary. Indeed, the illustrious Girolamo Mercuriale and Girolamo Capodivacca would disagree, advising instead in their report to the Venetian government that neither persons nor merchandise should be sent to the lazzaretto, and, furthermore, that it should be publicly declared that there was no plague in Venice.[12] Unfortunately, their assessment that the outbreak was a limited and far less dangerous "pestilential fever" was soon discredited by a rapidly mounting death rate. "It was hoped that in the opinion of the Paduan physicians [the disease] was not plague," the pope's representative in Venice, Giovan Battista Castagna, would report in July, "but now they are certain and in great fear because of a hundred deaths in a single day."[13] The Health Office's full prerogatives and protocols were reinstated, while the professors found themselves confined under quarantine. However, Mercuriale would continue to justify Capodivacca's and his own original diagnosis as accurate, by claiming that the outbreak had only subsequently developed into true plague.[14]

As many as one in every two Venetians may have fallen sick over the course of the epidemic of 1575–77 and more than half of those — a total of more than 50,000 people — were killed, a death rate estimated at approximately 28%.[15] Such staggering mortality served to reinforce the widespread conviction which had surrounded plagues since at least the Black Death, that outbreaks were ultimately supernatural scourges that could not possibly be controlled by terrestrial interventions alone. As a result, Venice would ultimately commend its fate to divine hands. In September 1576, the Venetian Republic formally beseeched Jesus Christ for rescue from the deadly affliction, pledging the first city-wide procession of thanksgiving since the fourteenth-century Black Death and additionally committing itself to the construction of a votive temple forever thereafter celebrating Venetians' liberation from the plague. Once the epidemic was officially declared over in July 1577, the results of this vow would be the city's annual festivities and splendid Palladian church dedicated to the Redeemer. Similarly, the government would turn to the Virgin Mary as *mediatrix* in the 1630–31 epidemic, pledging an annual votive commemoration to Santa Maria della Salute (Holy Mary of Health) and erecting a magnificent basilica in her name, designed by Baldassare Longhena.

During much of the sixteenth century, plague in Venice may have seemed like it was more or less under control. Since serious epidemics were becoming increasingly rare, the efforts of the Venetian Provveditori alla Sanità appeared to be successful, as sixteenth-century physician Bernardino Tomitano had claimed, for they "drive the plague not merely from one city, but from the [entire] world."[16] However, the devastating outbreaks of

FIG. 12
JEAN-JACQUES MANGET, *A Physician Dressed in Protective Plague Costume*, 1721. London, Wellcome Library

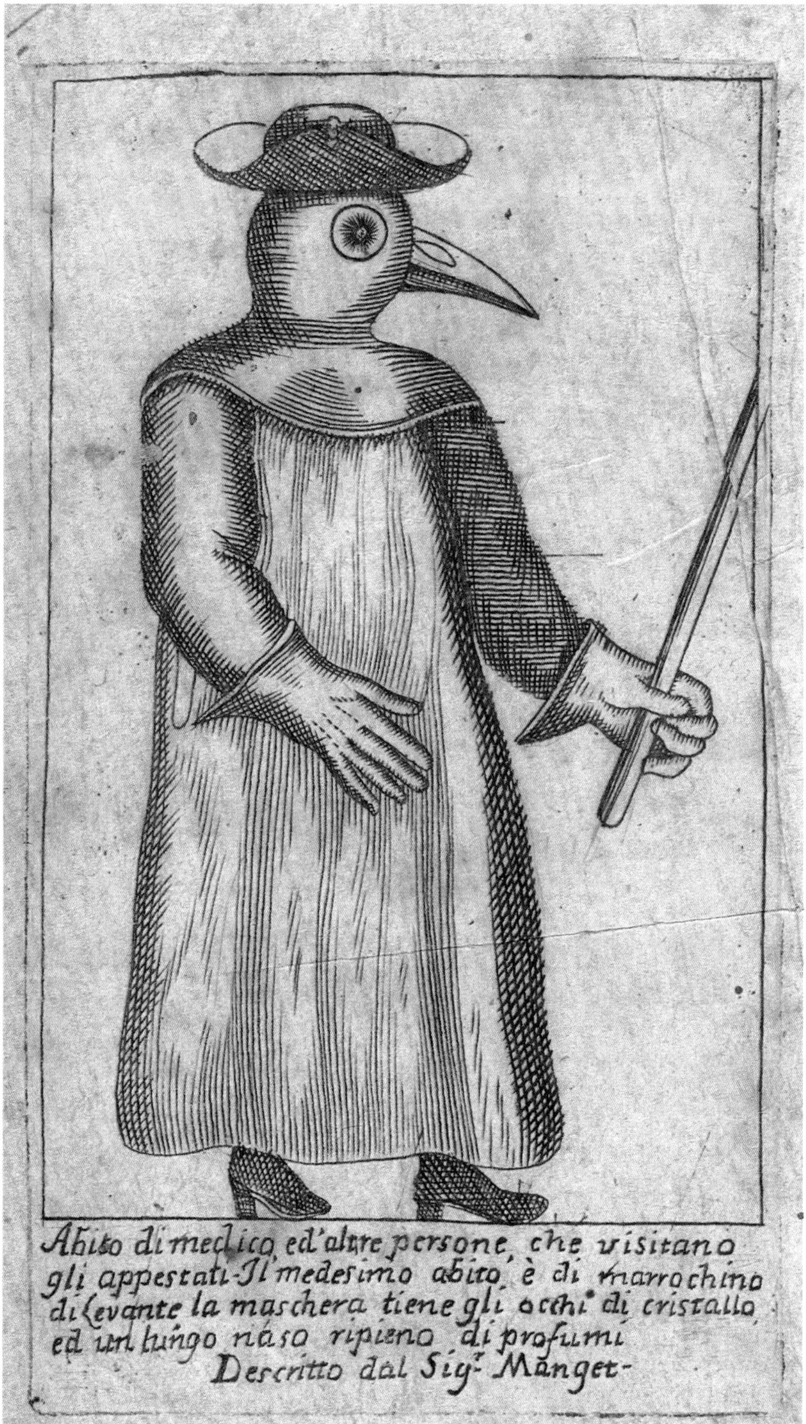
Abito di medico ed'altre persone, che visitano
gli appestati-Il medesimo abito, è di marrochino
di Levante la maschera tiene gli occhi di cristallo
ed un lungo naso ripieno di profumi
Descritto dal Sig.r Manget-

FIG. 12

1575–77 and 1630–31 served as correctives to any such premature hubris. In particular, the shock of the former sparked a crucial shift in European plague discourse, as an explosion of plague tracts appeared over the course of just four years. Accounting for nearly half of all plague tracts printed during the entire sixteenth century, these publications would expand plague literature from learned to lay, from Latin to the vernacular, and from the medical to the lyrical.[17] But, above all, this historically unprecedented flood of words memorialized the early modern struggle to comprehend and manage the intricate, vulnerable relationships between urban geography, human bodies, socio-economic lifestyles, the environment, trade, and even God's will, all of which possessed the potential to give rise to epidemics in an age of pestilence.

NOTES

1 Richard John Palmer, "The Control of Plague in Venice and Northern Italy, 1348-1600" (PhD diss., University of Kent at Canterbury, 1978), 328–37.

2 Since retrospective diagnosis is a fraught endeavor, debate persists regarding the identity of the infection which decimated mid-fourteenth century Europe, not to mention whether or not it may have recurred as often as "true plague" was subsequently cited in the historical record.

3 Despite the fact that today bubonic plague does not manifest exactly as did the original Black Death, the general consensus of most paleopathologists and historians of medicine seems to be that a variant of the same *Yersinia pestis* bacillus was nevertheless most likely responsible. Paul Slack, *Plague: A Very Short Introduction* (Oxford and New York, 2012), 7.

4 Whenever the quarantine system was activated, individuals evidencing symptoms were sent to the island of Santa Maria di Nazareth — now called the Lazzaretto Vecchio — where they would be treated in the plague hospital until their condition improved or else they succumbed to the disease. Persons who regained their health would then be transferred to the more distant Lazzaretto Nuovo near the island of Sant'Erasmo in the northern lagoon together with those who had been exposed to the infected but were as yet asymptomatic. Such individuals included not only residents but also merchants or travelers arriving from plague-afflicted areas, together with their possessions or wares, which would be aired out or fumigated there in order to try to disinfect them. Anyone who subsequently sickened would find themselves back at the Lazzaretto Vecchio, while those who did not develop any signs of infection within the allotted time would be permitted to enter the city proper.

5 Bruno Cecchetti, "La medicina in Venezia nel 1300," *Archivio Veneto*, n.s. 13, no. 26 (1883): 251–70.

6 Our current understanding of the etiology of bubonic plague originated only with the isolation of the *Y. pestis* bacillus in the late nineteenth century and, as a result, there was no awareness of the role of rodents' fleas as vectors in the spread of the disease during the Renaissance. Schools of thought regarding the apparent susceptibility of impoverished populations to the plague could focus on issues of geographical mobility or immobility (that is, when they may have been forced to travel through plague-infested areas as refugees or else were unable to afford to flee cities for the more salubrious countryside during urban epidemics) or, alternatively, upon their frequently unhealthy lifestyles and constitutions. Both considerations could be addressed by a poor hospital that provided improved nutrition and care for their physical health while segregating this potentially

infectious demographic from the general population.

7 Nancy G. Siraisi, *Medieval and Early Renaissance Medicine* (Chicago and London, 1990), 128; Samuel K. Cohn, Jr., *Cultures of Plague: Medical Thinking at the End of the Renaissance* (Oxford, 2010), 1 & 25–32.

8 Fracastoro would in fact coin the very term "syphilis" for what had up to that point been most commonly called the "French Disease" in his 1530 medico-mythological poem of the same name.

9 Girolamo Fracastoro, translated in Charles and Dorothea Singer, "The Scientific Position of Girolamo Fracastoro," in *Annals of Medical History*, Volume 1, ed. Francis R. Packard (New York, 1918), 27.

10 Michelle A. Laughran, "Medicating With or Without 'Scruples': The 'Professionalization' of the Apothecary in Sixteenth-Century Venice," *Pharmacy in History* 45, no. 3 (2003): 95–107.

11 While the origin of the English idiom is difficult to document, certainly the plague doctor wearing such "rose-colored glasses" might have had reason for optimism, not least because the plague mask would have functioned much as a modern surgical mask and safety goggles, protecting from pneumonic forms of plague or other droplet-disseminated concurrent infections, while the waxed robes and long gloves would have helped shield the wearer from infected fleas.

12 ASVe, *Secrete*, reg. 95, 19r-20r (20 June 1576) & 40r-46v (11 July 1576).

13 Giovan Battista Castagna, quoted in Palmer 1978, 253, note 2.

14 Cohn 2010, 167.

15 Jane L. Stevens Crawshaw, *Plague Hospitals: Public Health for the City in Early Modern Venice* (New York, 2012), 12, 178.

16 Bernardino Tomitano, *Consiglio dell'eccell. M. Bernardino Tomitano sopra la peste di Vinetia l'anno MDLVI* (Venice, 1556), 3r.

17 "The plague of 1575–8 gave rise to an explosion in plague poetry, which before 1575 had been rare [...]" (Cohn 2010, 25, 294).

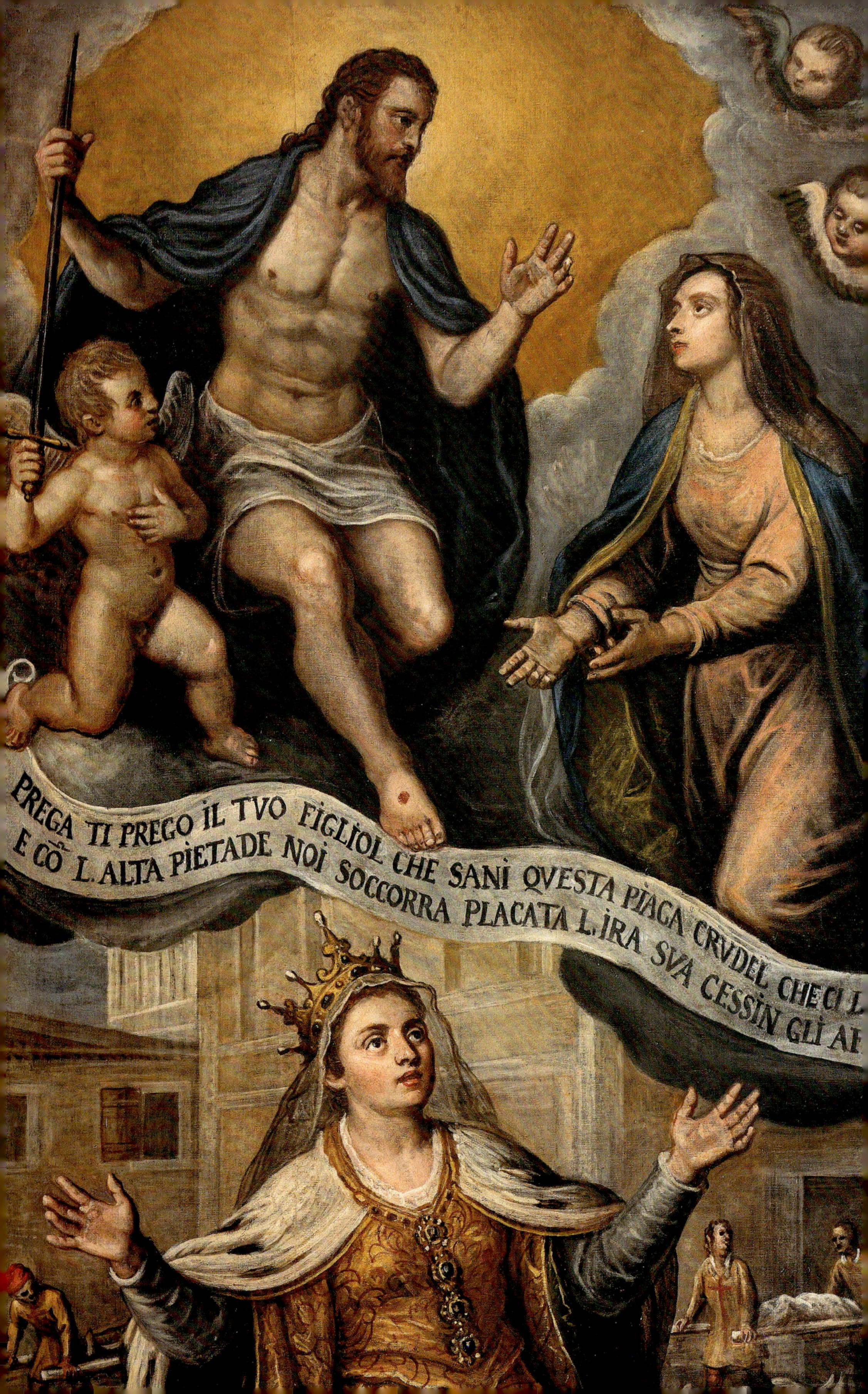
PREGA TI PREGO IL TVO FIGLIOL CHE SANI QVESTA PIAGA CRVDEL CHE CI L
E CŌ L. ALTA PIETADE NOI SOCCORRA PLACATA L.IRA SVA CESSIN GLI AF

DOMENICO TINTORETTO AND THE 1630–31 PLAGUE

Jennifer Gear

IN SUMMER 1630, a terrible outbreak of plague struck Venice. Between the disease's eruption in June 1630 and the Senate's declaration that the city was plague-free in November 1631, a third of the population, some 46,000 residents, had perished.[1] Domenico Tintoretto understood the danger, having survived the last devastating epidemic in the city in 1575–77. In October 1630, as plague deaths spiked, the artist prepared his will with a notary, aware of his mortality and advanced age during this public health crisis.[2]

Major plague epidemics affected all aspects of life in early modern Venice. The city's state-enforced quarantine and decontamination procedures, supported by the continuous operation of its two lazzaretti, were among the most sophisticated medical responses to plague in Europe during the sixteenth and seventeenth centuries.[3] Despite Venice's rigorous sanitation efforts and its isolation and treatment of plague victims, the 1630–31 outbreak was one of the worst in the city's history. To combat the disease spiritually and foster a sense of hope, Venetian residents honored the city's saints and holy protectors through public prayers, processions of sacred relics, and the commission of works of art that would represent their faith and appeals for protection.

Since plague's first appearance in Western Europe during the so-called Black Death of 1347–53, visual art played a central role in facilitating prayers and depicting the collective piety of congregations and confraternities. In the early modern period, plague art developed a set of genre-defining iconographies and conventions for depicting the disease. Patrons commissioning plague-themed works in Venice had expectations related to decorum, tradition, and the imaging of their own identities in relation to pestilence.

In 1631, while the epidemic raged in the city, Domenico Tintoretto was hired to create a plague painting for congregation members at San Francesco della Vigna in the Castello *sestiere*.[4] This votive work, *Venice Supplicating the Virgin to Intercede with Christ to End the Plague* (cat. 7), exemplifies plague art's varied functions in seventeenth-century Venice. It also offers a glimpse into Domenico's working methods. A preparatory sketch on paper created in the early stages of this project reveals that Domenico made striking changes to the work between the initial design and its final realization (fig. 13).[5] In place of the donor portraits at the bottom of the finished painting, the *modello* features an array of naked plague corpses, strewn at the knees of Venice personified.

It is unclear why Domenico adopted such radical changes to his painting's design, though there are several possibilities. The patrons — ostensibly the two women pictured in the work — may have objected to the graphic imagery. They have not been identified, nor have documents related to the commission been preserved, leaving stipulations for the work speculative. However, the significant difference between the iconography of the sketch and that of the final work reveals something of their preferences. The patrons may have requested less provocative imagery better suited to the painting's long-term use after the end of the epidemic. They may also have wanted their likenesses included to represent their status in the community and to aid them in obtaining greater protection from plague through the proximity of their portraits to the images of sacred figures pictured above. As a votive work, this painting petitioned Christ and the Virgin, giving form to the prayers offered in exchange for deliverance from the epidemic.

A banner unfurls diagonally across Domenico's painting, which reads: "Pray for me, I pray to your son for health, with the highest pity give aid to us against this evil wound that devours us — placate his wrath, ceasing our sighs."[6] This text separates the composition into two distinct registers: Venice in peril below, and the heavens above the city, where Christ, the Virgin, and angels have materialized. The clouds that give shape to this celestial realm dip just below the banner, touching the outstretched fingers of the personification of Venice, suggesting that salvation is attainable in even the direst of circumstances. Crowned and dressed in rich brocade and the ermine stole of the doge, the allegory of Venice embodies the protective power of the state and its inviolability. She is the city's primary intercessor and serves as an analogue to the Virgin. Their bodies are oriented toward one another, with a reciprocity magnified by their hand gestures. The Lion of Saint Mark crouches at Venice's knees, his eyes fixed on her with the reverence of a devoted dog. A "PAX" sign at his chest calls for peace in the city and references the legend in which an angel speaks to Mark on his initial arrival in Venice: "Peace be upon you, O Mark, my Evangelist."[7] This prophecy, in which God foretold of Saint Mark's return to Venice, was used as justification for the removal of the saint's body from Alexandria in 828 and its relocation to Venice.[8] Finally, Venice's extended arms call attention to the dangerous conditions in the city. Beneath each hand, tiny *pizzegamorti* are at work — body clearers carrying stretchers, collecting plague victims for disposal. The city is empty except for this macabre activity, heightening a sense of desolation.

While this characterization of Venice is unsettling, Domenico's initial representation of the city is terrifying. In the *modello*, the infected bodies of plague victims fill a third of the composition. They tip toward viewers and overwhelm the allegorical Venice kneeling beside them. A prominent "X" appears at the center of the sketch above Venice's arm, representing the boarded-up door of a house whose residents have either succumbed to

CAT. 7
DOMENICO TINTORETTO, *Venice Supplicating the Virgin to Intercede with Christ to End the Plague*, 1631

FIG. 13
DOMENICO TINTORETTO, sketch for *Venice Supplicating the Virgin to Intercede with Christ to End the Plague*, c. 1630–31. Princeton, Princeton University Art Musem, donation of Frank Jewett Mather Jr.

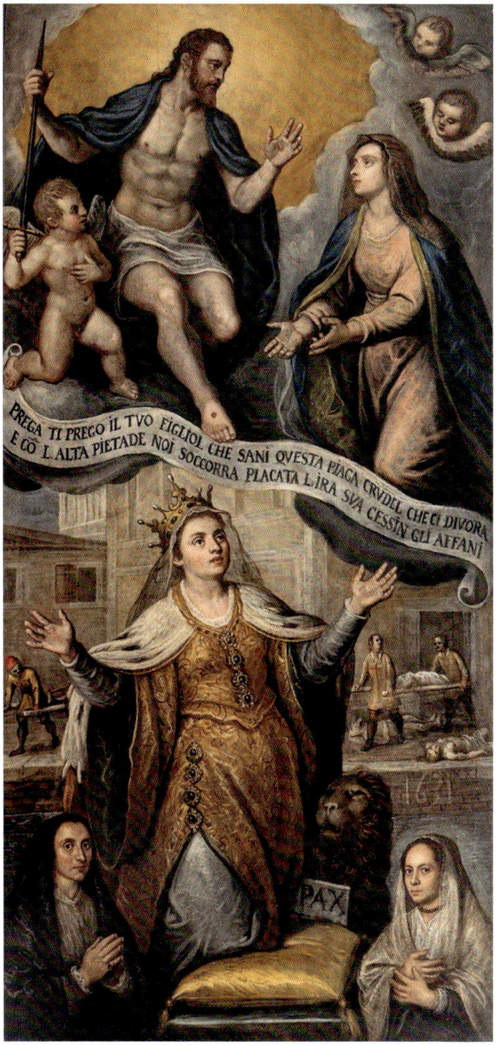
PREGA TI PREGO IL TVO FIGLIOL CHE SANI QVESTA PIAGA CRVDEL CHE CI DIVORA
E CŌ L ALTA PIETADE NOI SOCCORRA PLACATA L IRA SVA CESSIN GLI AFFANI
PAX

CAT. 7

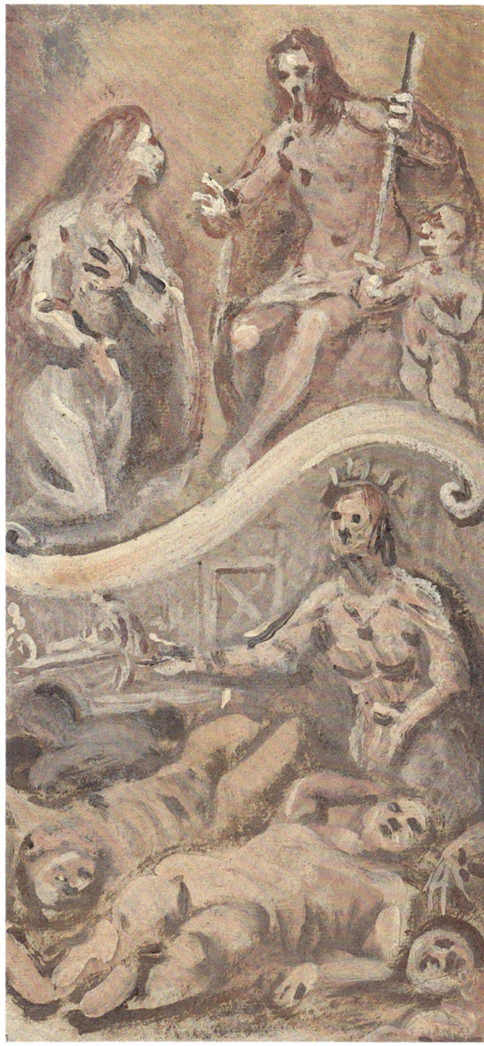

FIG. 13

plague or been sequestered in quarantine. Body clearers also haul victims on stretchers in this preparatory sketch, though the foreground corpses lessen these workers' disturbing potential. The Virgin, Christ, and a putto holding Christ's sword are represented similarly between *modello* and final painting, with one conspicuous difference that affects the entire composition: they appear in mirror image. Though creating drawings in reverse was common practice in the development of designs for print media, this appears not to be the case with Domenico's drawing. The composition's reversal between sketch and finished work reflects instead the painter's idiosyncratic method of settling on a successful composition, which is evident in other preparatory drawings he produced.[9] The portrayal of Christ holding the blade of his sword is unusual iconography that relates to the pictorial tradition of aligning pestilence with bodily mortification. Christ or God the Father are sometimes shown wielding arrows or a sword with which to strike humanity. Christ's staying of the weapon indicates he will grant the Virgin's plea for succor, and can be linked to the band of text that refers to plague as a wound.

In addition to representing the spiritual worth of congregation members at San Francesco della Vigna, *Venice Supplicating the Virgin to Intercede with Christ to End the Plague* may also have been used as a processional banner, carried outside the church during the epidemic in 1631. Seventeenth-century guidebooks indicate that this painting was not included in any of the church's private chapels, nor did it serve as an altarpiece, raising the question of how this painting was originally used.[10] The banner of text offers a clue. James Moore has noted that the prayer on Domenico's work matches phrasing found in litanies composed by Monteverdi while he was musical director at the Basilica di San Marco in 1630.[11] These litanies were performed during the weekly procession of a miracle-working image, the *Madonna Nicopeia*, around the Piazza San Marco during the epidemic. The imagery evoked by the motet aligns with the painting: "O happy portal, we cry to you [...] we sigh to you [...]/ She who is a secure link between men and God [...]."[12] In addition, an oration given by Doge Nicolò Contarini during the plague repeats this trope. Domenico was certainly aware of these sacred performances, and the closeness of the shared metaphors may indicate he created his votive painting to harmonize with State-organized prayers.

NOTES

1 P. Preto, "Le grandi pesti dell'età moderna: 1575-1577 e 1630-1631," in *Venezia e la peste: 1348-1797*, ed. O. Pugliese (Venice: Marsilio, 1979), 123–56, exhibition catalogue (Venice, Palazzo Ducale, 1979–1980); P. Ulvioni, *Il gran castigo di Dio: Carestia ed epidemie a Venezia e nella Terraferma, 1628-1632* (Milan: Franco Angeli Libri, 1989), 72–6.

2 Domenico's 1630 will is transcribed in E. March Phillips, *Tintoretto* (London: Methuen & Co., Ltd., 1911), 153–4.

3 For more on plague and Venice's *lazzaretti*, see R. Palmer, *The Control of Plague in Venice and Northern Italy, 1348-1600* (PhD diss. University of Kent at Canterbury), 1978; N.E. Vanzan Marchini (ed.), *Venezia e i lazzaretti mediterranei* (Mariano del Friuli: Edizioni della Laguna), 2004, exhibition catalogue (Venice, Biblioteca Nazionale Marciana, April 1-June 13 2004); J.L. Stevens Crawshaw, *Plague Hospitals: Public Health for the City in Early Modern Venice*, (Farnham, Surrey: Ashgate), 2012.

4 Pugliese 1979, 260–1; F. Ilchman, *Italian Master Drawings from the Princeton University Art Museum* ed. L.M. Giles, L. Markey, and C. Van Cleave (Princeton, NJ: Princeton University Art Museum, 2014), 121–4.

5 Ilchman 2014, 121–4.

6 In the vernacular, "Prega ti prego il tuo figliol che sani questa piaga crudel che ci divora/e con l alta pietade noi soccorra placata l ira sua cessin gli affani."

7 In Latin, "Pax tibi Marce Evangelista meus."

8 See David Rosand, *Myths of Venice: The Figuration of a State.* (Chapel Hill, London: University of North Carolina Press, 2001), 47–95.

9 Paola Rossi, "Per la grafica di Domenico Tintoretto, II," *Arte Veneta*, 38 (1984), 57–17; Michiaki Koshikawa, "I disegni di Domenico Tintoretto," *Arte Veneta*, 47 (1996), 56–69.

10 Marco Boschini, *Le minere della pittura* (Venice: 1664), 200–1; Pietro Antonio Pacifico, *Cronica veneta* (Venice: 1697), 185.

11 James Moore, "*Venezia favorita da Maria*: Music for the Madonna Nicopeia and Santa Maria della Salute," *Journal of the American Musicological Society*, 37 (Summer 1984), 332–6.

12 Ibid., 334.

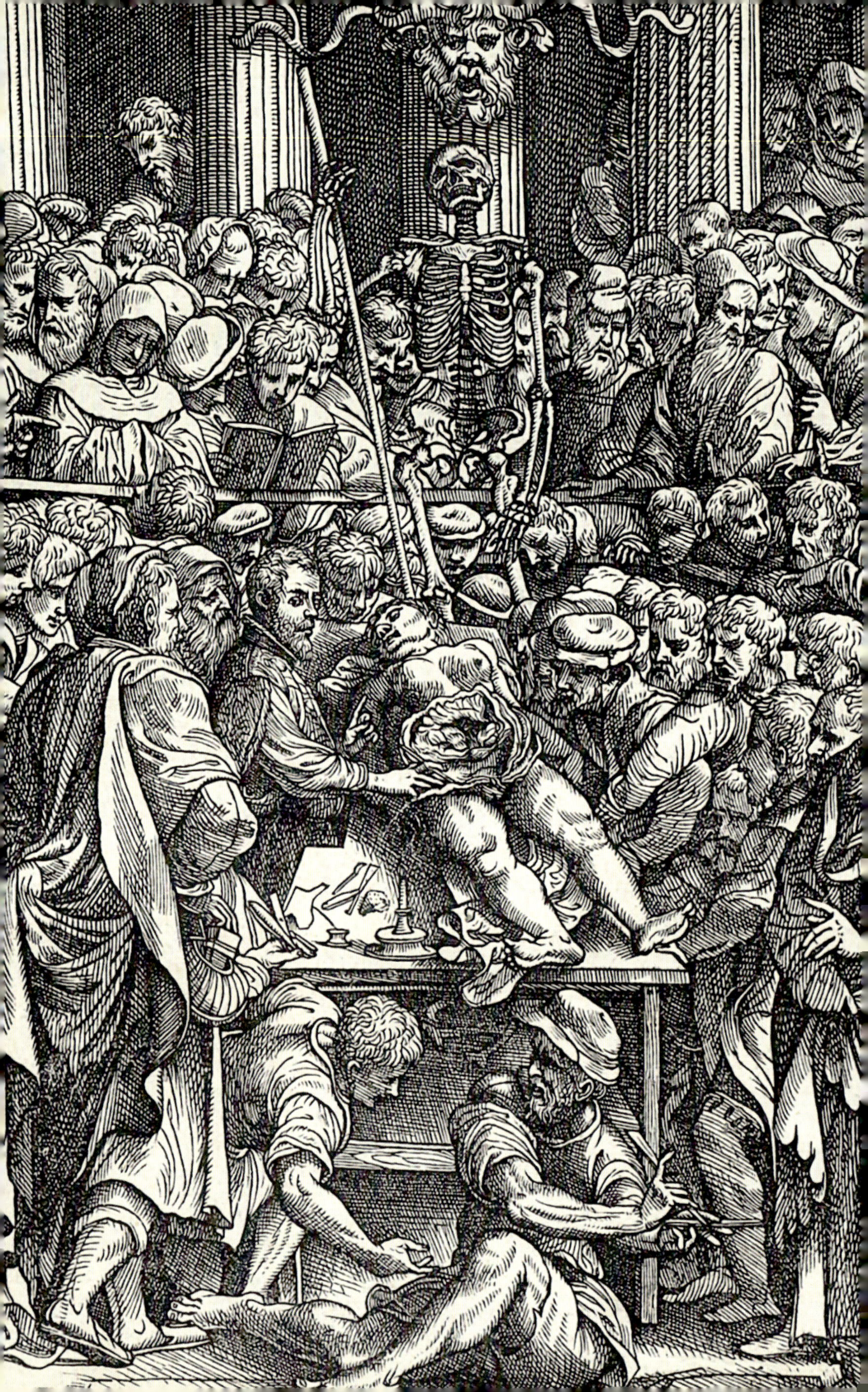

ANIMATING THE BODY: THE ROLES AND REASONS FOR ANATOMICAL STUDY IN THE RENAISSANCE

Cynthia Klestinec

> What could be more useful to a physician for the treatment of war-wounds, for extraction of missiles, for excision of bones, for [treatment of] dislocations, fractures with ulcerations [...] than to know accurately all the parts of the arms and legs, and all, not so much of the internal as of the external parts of the shoulders and back, breast and ribs, abdomen, neck, and head?[1]

IN THE SECOND CENTURY AD, Galen articulated this idea, which has become so basic, so fundamental to modern medicine, that it would be difficult to find a physician or a surgeon today who did not share it. This idea, however, was not immediately embraced as the most important rationale for human dissection. Rather, it ascended to prominence over time and through a complex set of historical processes.

In the Renaissance, the study of anatomy was pursued for a variety of reasons, not only because of its usefulness to the practice of medicine. Indeed, Galen himself offered two other motivations for undertaking dissections and acquiring anatomical knowledge. Anatomical study was important not only for the physician but also for the natural philosopher, "who loves knowledge for its own sake" and "values it only to demonstrate that Nature does naught in vain." And, lastly, both physicians and natural philosophers would find that anatomy provides "data" or experiences useful "for investigating a function, physical or mental," though some functions would be "of greater moment to natural philosophers than to physicians, both for pure knowledge and to show how the artifice of Nature is perfectly worked out in every part."[2] These additional uses presumed a teleological understanding of nature, and in the sixteenth century, they were pursued by natural philosophers at universities, that is, professors who sought to understand the nature of the body and its capacities. They were viewed as more important, for a time, than the uses that physicians and surgeons made of anatomy for treating their patients' wounds or attempting to cure their diseases.

Like today, the dissection of human and animal corpses is a special exercise, regulated by different entities or institutions, moderated by various individuals, mediated often by visual materials. Today, these include not only pictures but also computer-generated scenarios where the viewer "flies" through the body.[3] The materials of dissection — the corpse and interactive media — are thus coordinated in complex ways.

Different forms of mediation were present from the very origins of human dissection in the Middle Ages. No longer obscure, the origins of

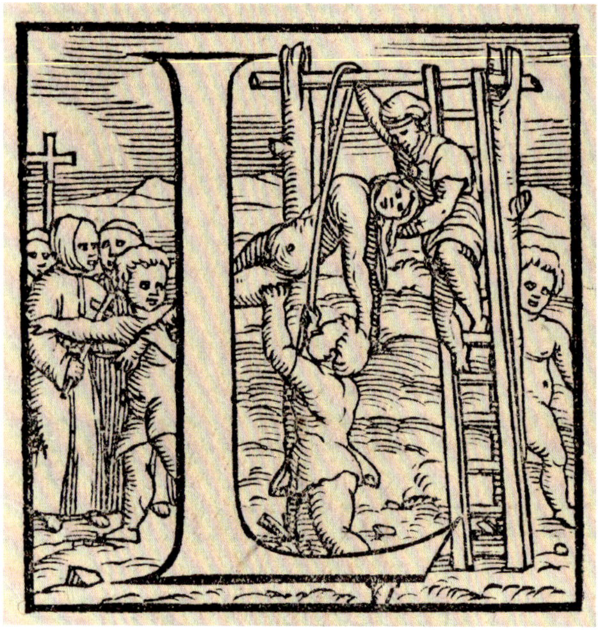

CAT. 38

human dissection for medical purposes in the West lie in the sacred spaces of nunneries, where the corpses of nuns were opened and scrutinized for signs of sanctity, signs which would be collected, described, and made significant through the processes of beatification.[4] Dissection as an investigative exercise was also connected to the practices of autopsy, when a corpse would be dissected and studied in order to ascertain the cause of death. An extension of the practice of autopsy was found in fourteenth-century Florence, when several patrician women, upon death, were autopsied in order to learn about their internal diseases, perhaps with the idea that treatment could be made available for their daughters, an early example of preventative health care.[5]

In medical schools across Europe, the practice of dissection evolved as a part of the medical curriculum.[6] With surprisingly little variation, the statutes for universities with medical curricula stipulated that one to two corpses a year would be supplied for dissection; and that these corpses were to be the bodies of criminals. Some of the decorated letters in Vesalius's *Fabrica* show putti removing the corpse from the scaffold of the execution (cat. 38). In addition, some statutes specify that these bodies had to be both criminal and foreign, probably to prevent a situation in which a student might encounter the dissection of his kin, perhaps a wayward uncle. These statutes thus imply the coordinated efforts of individuals and institutions: the university and its administration as well as religious and civic officials, who were involved in the juridical process. The coordinated involvement of the Church and the

CAT. 38
ANDREAS VESALIUS,
Andreae Vesalii Bruxellensis, … De humani corporis fabrica…,
Basel, 1555

state helps to correct the view that the Church opposed science in this period. This misunderstanding is a vestige of nineteenth-century accounts of the development of science, for in actuality, as religious history, the statutes of the university, and a wealth of civic archival material show, religious, political, and educational institutions worked together to provide anatomists, every year, with bodies for dissection. These institutions played a critical role in the medical and scientific developments of the period that we now call the Scientific Revolution. Indeed, those developments were grounded in the resources and character of those institutions.

The annual dissections took place in January and February. These were the coldest months of the year, which slowed the processes of decay and putrefaction. These annual events took place in temporary spaces, makeshift theaters with scaffolded seating, and, eventually, in more impressive permanent theaters. In Padua, the permanent theater, built in 1594–95, was described as "elegantly crafted" and "splendidly built"; it reflected the "glory" of Venice "no less than did the circus games and gymnasiums of antiquity." Descriptions such as these emphasize the theater's magnificence and its theatrical potential.[7]

Before permanent anatomy theaters were built, beginning in the 1580s, anatomy textbooks often featured dissection scenes and, increasingly throughout the sixteenth century, elaborate architecture framing those scenes as performative. As Andrea Carlino has explained, these scenes were both didactic and a ritualized demonstration of academic knowledge.[8] In the anatomy scene of Johannes de Ketham's text (cat. 33), the professor of anatomy stands behind a lectern, reading aloud a passage from a source; the *ostensor* would listen to the professor and likely translate the Latin for the dissector as he showed the dissector where to cut the body. The ritualized demonstration reasserted the authority of the source text rather than promoting the evidence of the body per se.

Adapting that tripartite organization, the frontispiece of Andreas Vesalius's *De humani corporis fabrica* (1543; cat. 36) features Vesalius himself next to the female corpse, which he has presumably dissected with his own hands, thereby collapsing the three roles — of professor, *ostensor*, and dissector — into one. The image also features an antiquated architectural frame surrounding the temporary theater. This has been compared to the courtyard of Palazzo del Bo at the University of Padua, where Vesalius taught, and to the recovery of classical sources on architecture, especially Vitruvius' *De architectura* and sixteenth-century editions of that text by Sebastiano Serlio among others. Indeed, architecture is a leitmotiv threaded through the *Fabrica*, not only in its name, which emphasizes the construction or fabrication of the human body, but also in the analogies that Vesalius borrowed from Galen, who stressed the similarities between the bones in a body and the frame of a house and the spine and keel of a

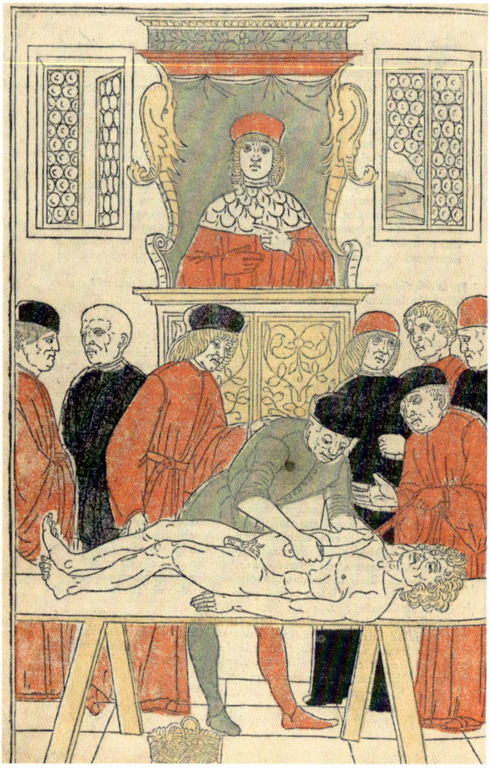

CAT. 33

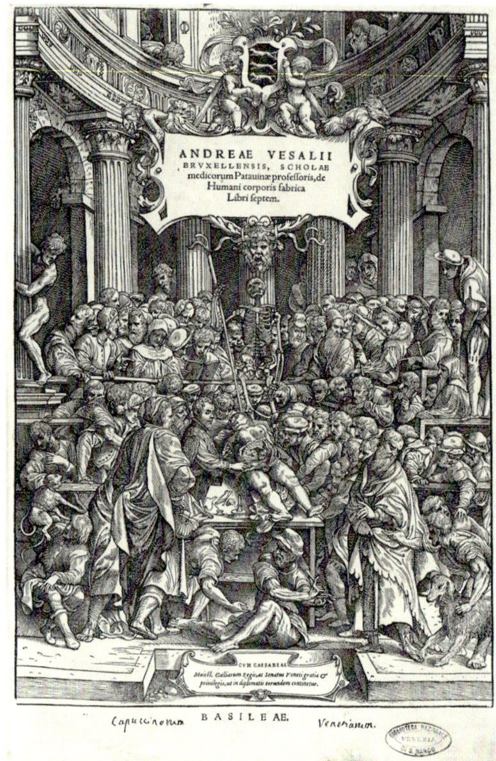

CAT. 36

CAT. 33
JOHANNES DE KETHAM, *Fasciculus medicinae*, Venice, 1493 [1494]

CAT. 36
ANDREAS VESALIUS, *Andreae Vesalii Bruxellensis, ... De humani corporis fabrica...*, Basel, 1543

ship, as well as the presence of classical ruins in the background to the text's illustrations of dissected bodies.

While Galen acknowledged several reasons for studying anatomy, medical students tended to be more focused on its usefulness for medical practice. In addition to the annual anatomy demonstration, there were dissections throughout the year that were attended by a smaller group of students. These "private" dissections, which took place at hospitals, apothecaries, and even the anatomist's home, could be focused not only on specific research questions but also on general anatomy useful to surgical interventions or even pathological inquiry.[9] In Padua, students complained that the main anatomist, Hieronymus Fabricius, did not provide them with a coherent or complete understanding of the general anatomy of the human body, that he attempted to "evade all things anatomical."[10] His anatomy demonstrations tended to focus on parts and groups of parts, such as the parts associated with the senses, or with locomotion, which were not only important to his research but which were also used to investigate and illustrate the (natural) philosophical dimensions of anatomy. Fabricius is associated with a series of anatomical oil paintings of dissected parts (cat. 10), which could serve

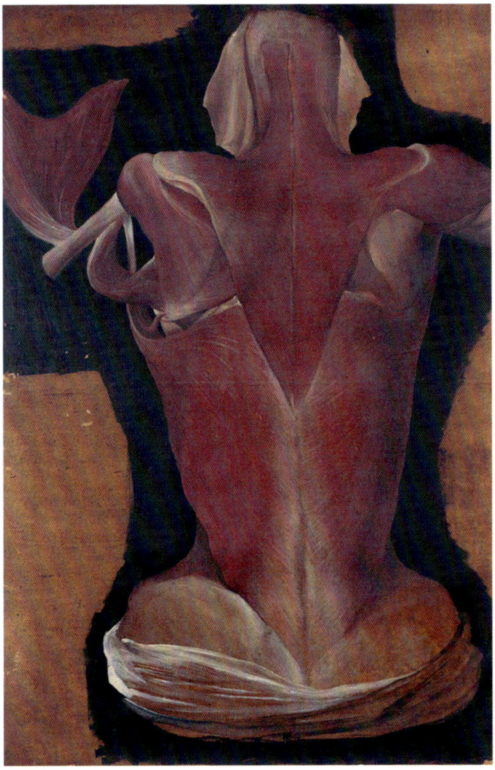

CAT. 10

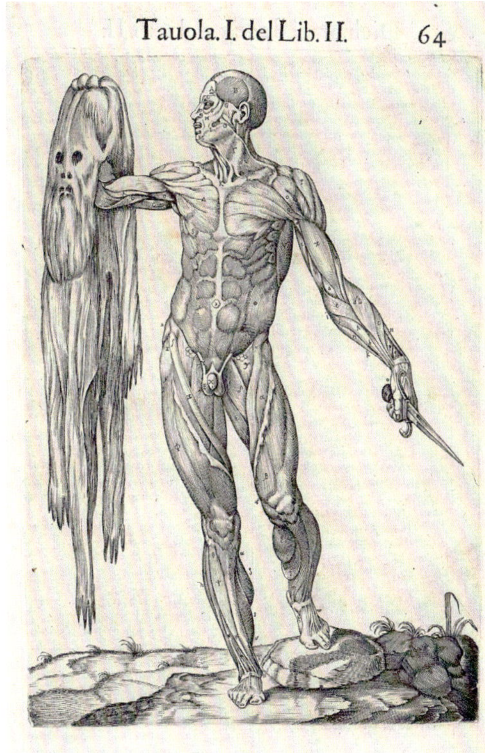

CAT. 39

students as enhanced study guides, as images to compare in the context of an actual dissection, and as initial steps in a fuller, philosophical account of, say, vision.[11] Intriguingly, the artist has used color to distinguish structures (something that printed images in books could not yet accomplish).

In Venice, the approach to the study of anatomy and human dissection tended to include more practical considerations. The Venetian College of Surgeons hosted annual anatomies as well as disputations and examinations for degrees and licenses. Many of its members were also professors in Padua: Alessandro Benedetti, Vittor Trincavella, Gabriele Falloppio, as well as, late in his career, Hieronymus Fabricius; and, in the seventeenth century, Santorio Santorio and Johann Veslingus were both members.[12] The College of Surgery provided medical students with additional instruction on anatomy that was both learned (coming from the Latinate tradition) and practical.

Similar to the university in Padua, the statutes for the College indicate that public anatomies were to take place annually; and the records of the college show that they happened more regularly in the second half of the sixteenth century. These events were held at the church of San Paternian, which no longer exists, and the church of Santo Stefano, among other

CAT. 10
HIERONYMUS FABRICIUS, *De anatomia musculorum totius corporis*, before 1619

CAT. 39
JUAN VALVERDE DE AMUSCO, *Anatomia del corpo humano...*, Venice, 1560

locations in Venice.[13] Anatomy lessons were attended not only by physicians and surgeons but also by barbers. In 1603, when the physician Fabio Glissenti was elected reader for the annual anatomy, the records of the college explain that even barbers needed this experience because:

> There are many barbers that treat [patients] in Venice and let blood, [and] many of them have never cut [bodies] nor seen the cutting in an anatomy of the human body, and so they do not know how the veins and the other parts of our body [go]; because of this, many errors are committed.[14]

In addition, public anatomies were important to the process of building a medical career. As Richard Palmer has explained, in the 1560s, the famous physician-surgeon Niccolò Massa testified on behalf of Zuata Francesco da Burano, who was then petitioning the doge to allow his son Giacomo to practice with him in the service of the Venetian Republic; Massa said that Giacomo was not only a doctor in the art of medicine, learned in philosophy and medicine, both physic and surgery, but also "a man of worth [*homo de valor*]."[15] Massa went on to say that this year, when the anatomy was held, "finding myself with him and discussing the anatomy, I saw and heard that Giacomo has a very good understanding of these matters." Massa's father was a physician, and he testified that Giacomo took his doctorate in the College in Venice and that the vote on him was unanimous. He continued by noting that Giacomo had "observed anatomies and also with his own hands has practiced privately with other doctors." The testimonies of Massa and his father suggest that while anatomical knowledge retained its practical purpose, it was also one of the criteria for judging a practitioner's suitability for membership into a medical elite, for Giacomo's appointment was subsequently confirmed by the Venetian Senate.

Not everyone, however, was convinced that attending an anatomy demonstration would translate into more effective practice or better outcomes. One sixteenth-century practitioner (who was not trained at the university), Leonardo Fioravanti (1517–88), acknowledged that we all wish to know the illnesses inside the body, "to know precisely how it happens that one suffers on the inside."[16] But, he cautions:

> I will say, ardently believing what I say is true, that I have never known a man who has seen so many anatomies of living human bodies as I have seen in different wars, where I have found myself; and yet I confess freely to not knowing these things; this estimation came not so much from my inability as from the fact that the thing itself is impossible to know.[17]

Such skepticism reminds us that an anatomical understanding of the body was not immediately viewed as essential to medicine, and that the ascendance of such an idea required anatomists, students, and medical practitioners to pursue the philosophical accounts of anatomy that explored the function of

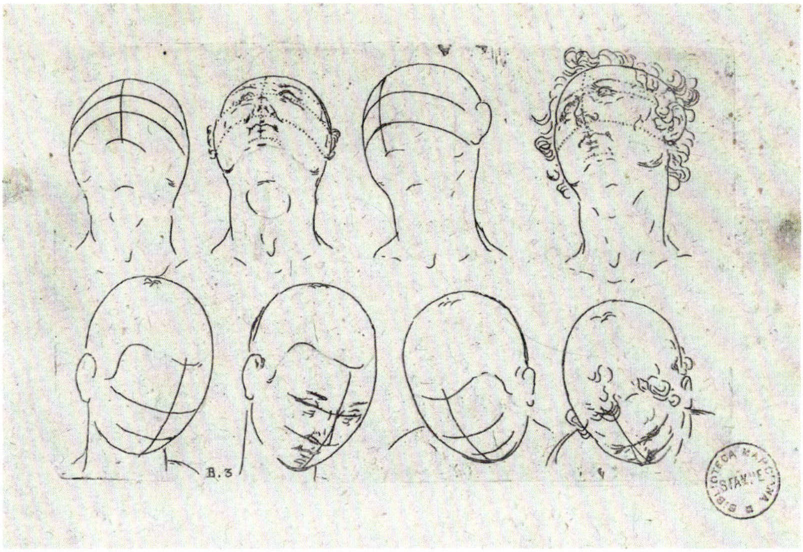

CAT. 59

parts in a state of health and in one of disease, and to insist on better practical applications of anatomy through the field of surgery.

Although the usefulness of anatomy was debated in both philosophical discussions and in practical, medical ones, the images associated with anatomy emphasize the importance of the dictum "know thyself" (*nosce te ipsum*). Self-knowledge generated an iconographical tendency to show cadavers in various stages of dissection displaying their own body parts. In his Vesalian edition of anatomy, Juan Valverde de Hamusco, a Spanish writer living in Rome and connected to its community of printers, included an image of a cadaver showing his own skin, removed (cat. 39). Echoing the flaying of Marsyas, also incorporated into Michelangelo's *Last Judgement*, the figure belies its own torture even as it reveals the system of muscles in the body. In the anatomy textbook of Iulius Caesar Casserius, who was a student of Hieronymus Fabricius, the muscled figure is shown pulling back his own skin, a flap, to reveal the muscles beneath. Casserius's figure, however vivified and visually compelling, recalls the earlier tradition of "flap anatomies." These were books that had flaps of paper that could be partially lifted in order to expose deeper, more internal anatomical structures. These kinds of artifacts emphasize the body's depth, its role as a container of parts and, perhaps more suggestively, the architecture of that container. Vesalius's *Epitome* was a part of this tradition of flap anatomies, where the flaps would be assembled by the user.

CAT. 59
ODOARDO FIALETTI,
Il uero modo et ordine...,
Venice, 1608

These visual trends also participated, however obliquely, in the traditions of artistic connoisseurship in the period. Casserius's images find visual counterparts in the drawing manuals of the same period, such as those by Odoardo Fialetti, Giacomo Franco, or Gasparo Colombina, which reveal studies of head shapes, angles and perspectives. Catherine Whistler has recently shown how these manuals (cat. 59), in addition to serving artists, were of interest to art collectors.[18] A similar interest might have been taken in anatomical texts, which could be lavishly illustrated, and even inspired some of Tommaso Giannotti Rangone's own collecting practices.[19]

The cultures of anatomy and dissection included philosophical and medical rationales for human dissection, as Galen had anticipated. In Venice, annual anatomy demonstrations engaged not only physicians but also educated surgeons and illiterate barbers. These events were orchestrated by religious, civic, and medical institutions. Moreover, public dissections bear witness to a broad range of questions about the secrets of the body and its sacred and scientific significance, questions that animated medical discussions and debates and the visual projects of the age, as well as, undoubtedly, patients' experiences of health and illness.

NOTES

1 *Galen On Anatomical Procedures*, trans. C. Singer (Oxford: Oxford University Press, 1956), 33.

2 Ibid., 34.

3 See, for example, the Visible Human Project: https://lhncbc.nlm.nih.gov/project/visible-human-project.

4 Katharine Park, *Secrets of Women: Gender, Generation and the Origins of Human Dissection* (New York: Zone Books, 2006).

5 Ibid.

6 On the medical curriculum, see M. McVaugh, *The Rational Surgery of the Middle Ages* (Florence: Sismel, 2006); and N.G. Siraisi, *Medieval and Early Renaissance Medicine: An Introduction to Knowledge and Practice* (Chicago: University of Chicago Press, 1990) and *Avicenna in Renaissance Italy: The Canon and Medical Teaching in Italian Universities After 1500* (Princeton: Princeton University Press, 1987). On the study of medicine in Padua, see G. Ongaro, "La medicina nello Studio di Padova e nel Veneto," in *Storia della cultura veneta: Dal primo quattrocentro al consilio di Trento*, Vol. 3, ed. G. Arnaldi and M.P. Stocchi (Vicenza: Neri Pozza, 1981), 75–113.

7 G.F. Tomasini, *Gymnasium Patavinum*, Vol. 31 (Udine: 1654), 79–81.

8 A. Carlino, *La fabbrica del corpo: libri e dissezione nel Rinascimento* (Turin: Einaudi, 1994), which was published in English as *Books of the Body: Anatomical Ritual and Renaissance Learning* (Chicago: University of Chicago Press, 1999).

9 C. Klestinec, *Theaters of Anatomy: Students, Teachers, and Traditions of Dissection in Renaissance Venice* (Baltimore: Johns Hopkins University Press, 2011).

10 *Atti della nazione germanica [Acta germanicae artistarum] 1577-1578*, ed. A. Favaro (Venice, 1911–12), Vol. 1, 132–33. See Klestinec, ibid.

11 On these oil paintings, see *Il teatro dei corpi: le pitture colorate d'anatomia di Girolamo Fabrici d'Acquapendente*, ed. M. Rippa Bonati and J. Pardo-Tomàs (Milan: Mediamed, 204), exhibition catalogue (Venice, Biblioteca Nazionale Marciana, December 17, 2004-May 18, 2005); particularly N. Siraisi's contribution, "*Historia, actio, utilitas*: Fabrici e le scienze della vita nel Cinquecentro," 63–73.

12 See F. Bernardi, *Prospetto Storico-Critico. Dell'origine, facoltà, diversi stati, progressi, e vicende del Collegio Medico-Chirurgico, e dell'Arte Chirurgica in Venezia* (1797) in *Dalla scienza medica alla pratica dei corpi: fonti e manoscritti marciani per la Storia della Sanità*, ed. N.E. Vanzan Marchini (Venice: Neriz Pozza, 1993), 77–162.

13 BNM, It.VII 2370 (9668), Cap XXXVI, 81, *De anatomia*. Between 1550 and 1605, the records indicate that anatomies took place in 1574, 1585, 1594, 1602, and 1603. See BNM, It.VII.2327-2335 (9721-9729) *Collegio medico chirurgico di Venezia: Atti* (1476-1805), Libro D: 1549-1628 (cc.171).

14 BNM, It.VII.2327-2335 (9721-9729) *Collegio medico chirurgico di Venezia: Atti* (1476-1805), Libro D: 1549-1628 (cc.171): 131r.

15 R. Palmer, "Physicians and Surgeons in Sixteenth-Century Venice," *Medical History* 23 (1979): 451–460, 458. See also R. Palmer, "Nicolò Massa, His Family and His Fortune," *Medical History* 25 (1981): 385–410; and, on the Paduan students who took degrees in Venice, *The Studio of Venice and Its Graduates in the Sixteenth Century* (Padua: Lint, 1983).

16 L. Fioravanti, *Dello specchio di scientia universale* (Venice: Valgrisi, 1564), 13–14.

17 Ibid.

18 C. Whistler, "Learning to Draw in Venice: The Role of Drawing Manuals," in *Rethinking Renaissance Drawings*, ed. U. Roman D'Elia (Montreal-Kingston-London-Chicago: McGill-Queen's University Press, 2015), 121–136.

19 On Rangone's professional career and collection, see S. Minuzzi's essay in this volume.

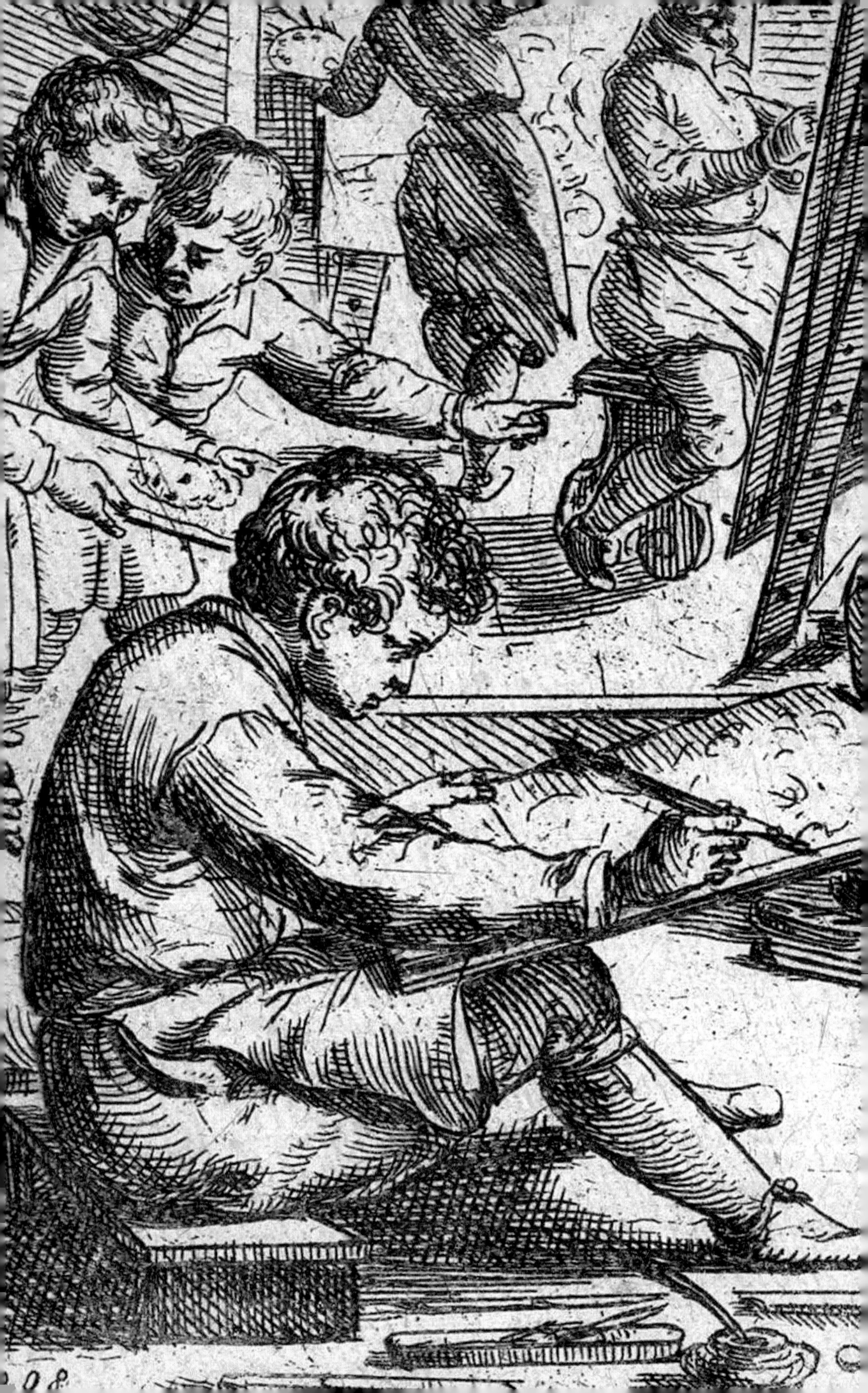

DOMENICO TINTORETTO'S LIFE-DRAWING: ANATOMY OF AN ARTISTIC REFORM

Gabriele Matino

LOCATED, ACCORDING TO Carlo Ridolfi's *Le maraviglie dell'arte*, in the "remotest part of the house,"[1] the Tintoretto studio must have been at the back of the small palazzo belonging to the Robusti family on Fondamenta dei Mori, a building that once adjoined Palazzo Mastelli del Cammello.[2] Ridolfi did not step foot into this out-of-the-way place until after the death of Jacopo Tintoretto (May 31, 1594), and long after his son Domenico had succeeded him as the head of the workshop. Having crossed the threshold, Ridolfi found himself in a room crammed with the sculptures Jacopo had accumulated over the years (cat. 59): from casts and replicas of ancient statues to models based on works of Michelangelo Buonarroti and other Florentine sculptors.[3] In all likelihood, Ridolfi already knew about this collection, but the drawings Domenico showed him must have had quite a different effect on the biographer: all at once, the origin of Tintorettesque aesthetics was revealed.

From his visit to the workshop, Ridolfi reconstructed the profile of an artist whose work, although inspired by Titian's use of color, found its constitutive principle in the practice of drawing. It was thanks to some drawings made "with charcoal and the colors of his father's dyes," the biographer informs us, that Jacopo had been entrusted to Titian's guidance while still a boy. A few days after his arrival in the workshop, it was this talent for drawing that alarmed the painter from Cadore, who, realizing that Jacopo "could become a skillful artist," decided to kick him out without much ceremony. Left without a teacher, it was by copying Michelangelo's statues that the young autodidact was able to develop his "strong and resolute manner"; at the same time, though, it was by studying from life — chiefly drawing models, but also cadavers whose skin he stripped off himself — that Jacopo gained an understanding of the "structure of the muscles." It was, Ridolfi concludes, the incessant practice of drawing that allowed Jacopo to achieve "the most difficult feat in art": dressing the imperfections of the human body in ideal beauty so as to "add to Nature's beauty with art."[4]

Given the crucial role drawing plays in his biography of Jacopo, it is surprising that Ridolfi makes no mention of it in his life of Domenico.[5] Ridolfi's omission is particularly startling in view of the fact that in his last will and testament (October 20, 1630), Domenico left his successor, Sebastiano Casser, 200 of his "sketches from life," to be chosen from among the far more numerous examples in his collection.[6] It is hard to believe that Domenico would have failed to show Ridolfi his drawings during the visit,

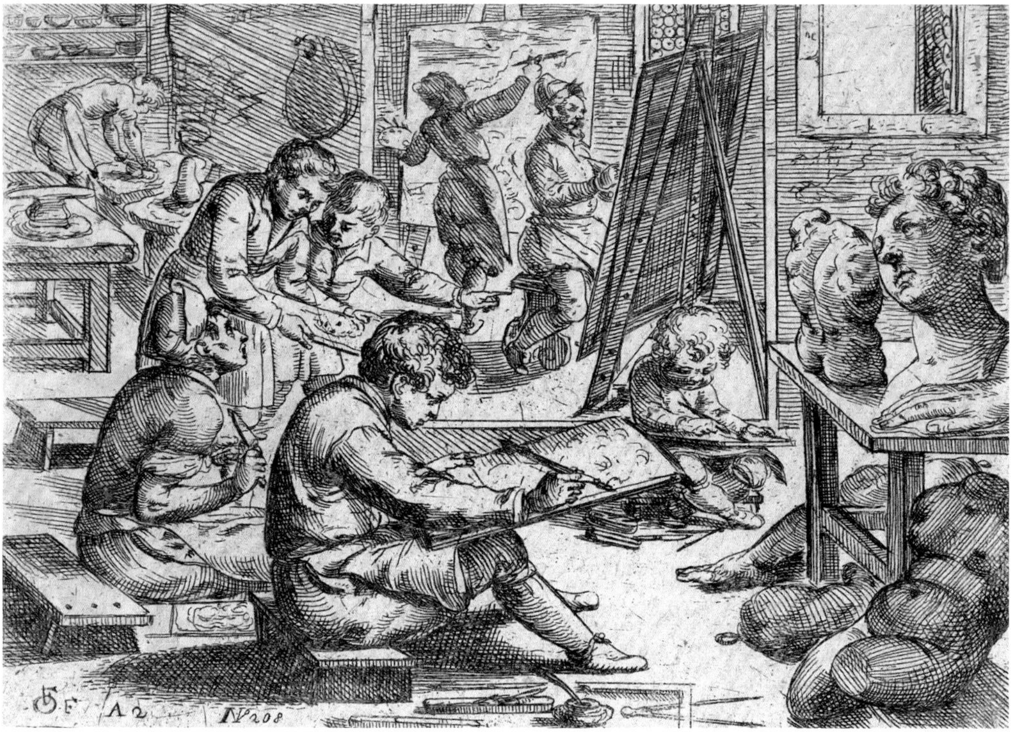

CAT. 59

so we must presume that there were deeper reasons for the biographer's silence. A clue can be found at the beginning of the text, where Ridolfi rebukes Domenico for "disdaining to continue on the true path" and straying from his father's manner.[7] To better understand how and why Domenico tried to free himself from his father's intimidating shadow, it will be helpful to look at his graphic output, which, as we shall see, contained the germ of an artistic reform that must have considerably troubled the artist's biographer.

Heir apparent to the family workshop, Domenico was trained in the art of drawing from an early age, so that he may learn his father's approach to graphic art and master his visual language.[8] The apprenticeship must have begun with the study of sculptural models, such as Michelangelo's *Samson and the Philistines*, of which Tintoretto possessed a copy in wax or clay: over sixty sketches have survived that can be assigned to Jacopo and his pupils. For the purposes of this argument, it is worth considering a folio in the Uffizi (Inv. 1069S, verso), now attributed to Domenico. While the hesitant execution reflects the young apprentice's lack of experience, the insertion on the margin of a sketch of one of his companions studying the same scuptural group is of considerable interest. It shows that in Tintoretto's workshop Michelangelo's models were studied in group sessions, and the different pupils' works were probably compared and carefully evaluated by the master.[9]

CAT. 59
ODOARDO FIALETTI,
Il uero modo et ordine...,
Venice, 1608

As well as exercises in the copying of statues, the lessons included life drawing. Among the sketches produced by Domenico in his youth there is a folio, now in the Pierpont Morgan Library in New York (fig. 15),[10] in which the pose of the model on the right, portrayed from the rear and resting on his left arm, which he places behind his back, seems to have been inspired by the pose of Michelangelo's *Dusk* for the Medici Chapels in Florence. The drawing shows how at this stage Domenico was trying to filter the lesson of Michelangelo's sculpture by imitating the rapid, broken lines that were typical of his father's style.

A pair of studies of a *Standing Nude Figure with a Ladder*, now in the Uffizi (fig. 14),[11] should be assigned to a later period: two snapshots of a session of life drawing in which a young model was observed from several points of view, as if he had been a sculpture. In contrast to the exercises on casts of Michelangelo sculptures, however, in these drawings Domenico attenuated the relief of the musculature and, following Jacopo's example, he opted for a more succinct and summary representation of the model's anatomy. The hasty execution reflects the nature of the session, which was no longer a teaching exercise, but a means of rapidly capturing poses and gestures that could be utilized in future compositions. Indeed, it is no coincidence that the two sketches were reused by Domenico both in the *Capture of Constantinople* for the Palazzo Ducale (after 1594)[12] and, as is proposed here, in the canvases for the cycle of scenes from the life of Saint Mark in the chapel of the Scuola Grande di San Marco (c. 1587–92). The reference is first of all to the *Standing Nude Figure with a Ladder* who, located by Domenico on the left of *Saint Mark Blessing the Venetian Islands* (cat. 2), appears to be in the act of lifting the boat's rudder, which has taken the place of the ladder in the drawing from life. The same figure reappears in the *Dream of Saint Mark* (cat. 1), now almost entirely covered by a green cloak and red cap. In the same cycle, finally, there is a striking similarity of pose between the *Standing Nude from Behind with Ladder* (Department of Prints and Drawings, Uffizi Galleries, Florence, Inv. 12951F) and one of the two Venetians carrying the body of the Evangelist (cat. 3).

The first signs of an artistic personality that was independent of his father's were already apparent in Domenico's graphic production of the 1580s. These years followed the return to Venice of Jacopo Palma il Giovane, whose quest for naturalism also entailed studies from life,[13] many of which have been confused with ones by Domenico.[14] Above all, in this period Agostino and Annibale Carracci made repeated stays in Venice, and their encounters with Domenico, who was roughly the same age, must have gone well beyond what is normally acknowledged by critics.[15] As early as 1582 the two painters, together with their cousin Ludovico, had founded the Accademia degli Incamminati in their hometown of Bologna. The leaders of the academy regarded the study of the nude figure as an activity of critical importance. As in the case of Domenico's drawing in the Morgan Library, the Carracci instructed their

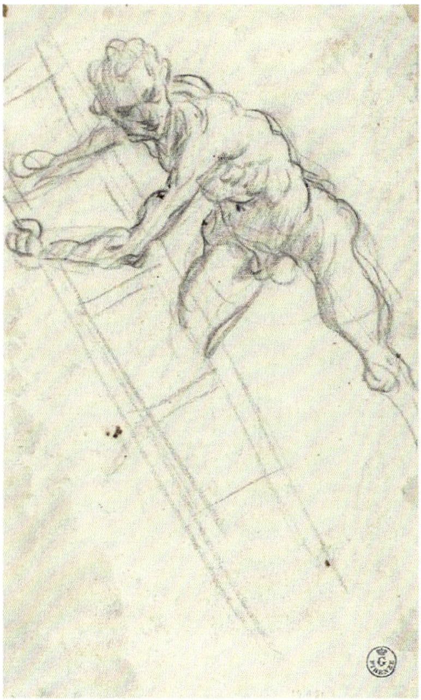

FIG. 14

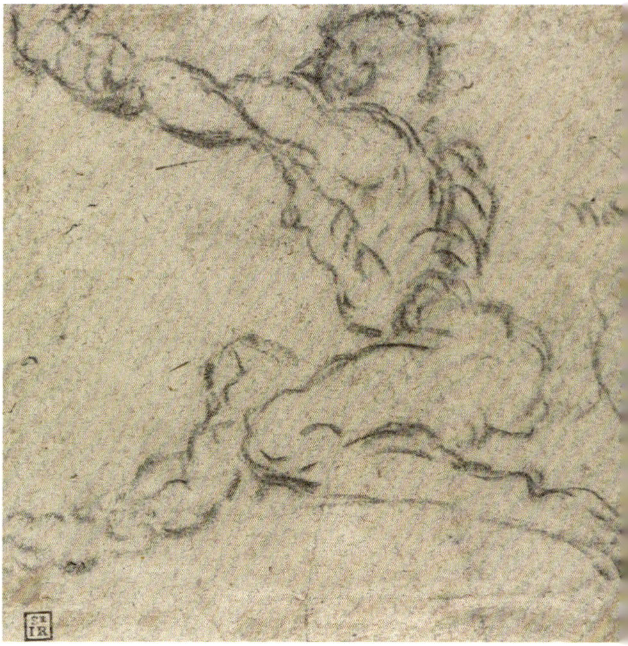

FIG. 15

FIG. 14
DOMENICO TINTORETTO (attrib.), *Standing Nude Figure with a Ladder*, c. 1580–90, Florence, Department of Prints and Drawings, Uffizi Galleries

FIG. 15
DOMENICO TINTORETTO (attrib.), *Two Seated Nude Figures*, recto, final quarter of the sixteenth century, New York, The Morgan Library & Museum. Acquired by Pierpont Morgan (1837–1913) in 1909

models to assume Michelangelesque poses, but, in contrast to what was done in Tintoretto's workshop, the result was a moderation of Buonarroti's monumentality, which was brought back into the sphere of the natural. In contrast to the artistic legacy of the great masters of the early sixteenth century, the Carracci's reform was to make nature, rather than art, the canon of reference.[16]

Domenico's first, timid foray in this direction can be discerned in some female nude studies in which the typically Tintorettesque handling of the outlines combines with a novel interest in realism. A clear example of this is provided by a drawing now in the Musée du Louvre (fig. 16) in which soft cross-hatching is used to convey the generous forms of a model reclining with sensual abandon. This study documents the educational nature of the sketch, especially if we consider the way Domenico has lingered over repeated anatomical details in the margins. Moreover, when the folio is compared with other examples in the Louvre (Inv. 7514r) and the Uffizi (Inv. 13001F),[17] it becomes clear that this and other drawings from life were used by the painter to study the pose of a *Sleeping Venus*, a theme that Domenico was to develop with surprising results.

It was only after Jacopo's death that reality became an aesthetic principle in Domenico's graphic work, in an increasingly conscious rejection of his father's manner. When singing Jacopo's praises, Ridolfi had celebrated the artist's realization that "strict imitation of nature was not enough, for nature

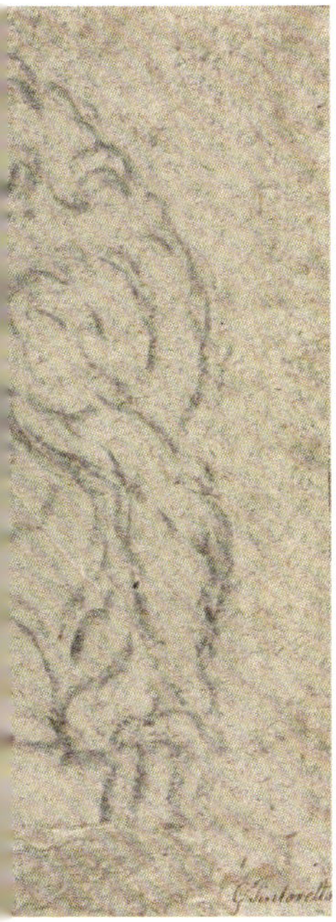

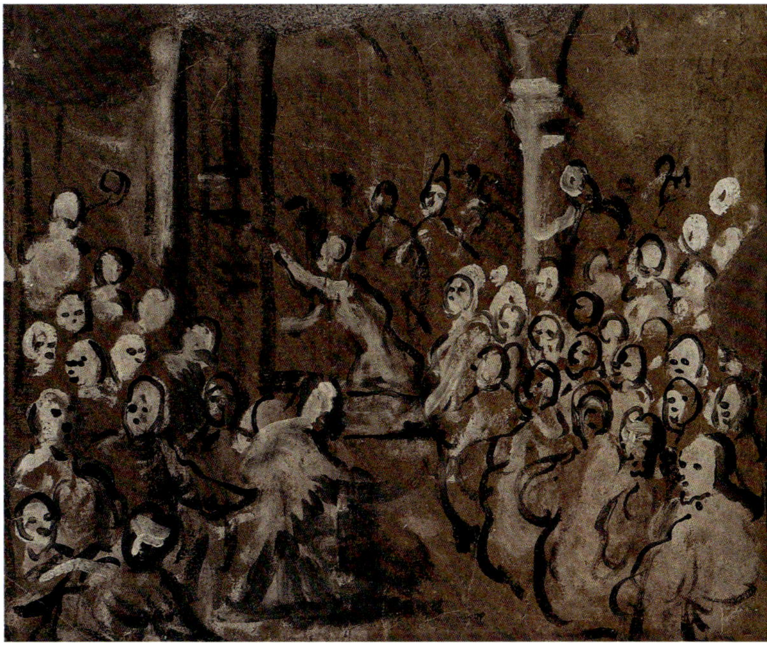

CAT. 11

produces mostly imperfect things." It was not that Tintoretto had not devoted himself to study from life, but he had chosen to set an idealizing filter over the imperfections of the human body, in order to produce a "contrived manner filled with much beauty."[18] When he became head of the Tintoretto workshop, Domenico decided to go down a different road.

Evidence for this comes from life studies at different stages of completion that are nevertheless uniform in their intentions. Among the numerous examples, it is worth mentioning those in the Metropolitan Museum (Inv. 1975.1.533-539) and at the Fondation Custodia in Paris (Inv. 1362), which can be dated to the first thirty years of the seventeenth century.[19] The sketches show Domenico intent on analyzing the female body, an exercise he had already practiced in the 1580s; this time, however, he preferred ungainly bodies to ideal forms. One of the most disconcerting examples (fig. 17) is that of a model with thinning hair, coarse and prominent features, and a body so ambiguous in its gender that some scholars have been induced to identify it as male. No less surprising, and indeed even more extreme in their results, are the studies (now in The Metropolitan Museum) of a model with a gnarled body, scrawny legs, and a belly swollen in pregnancy, which Domenico depicted with a degree of objectivity unknown to his contemporaries. Although the poses he asked the models to assume still recall the theme of the *Sleeping Venus*, it is the deglamorizing unattractiveness of their bodies that indicated the artistic process that was underway. In surprising affinity with

CAT. 11
DOMENICO TINTORETTO, Sketch for the *Miracle of the Ring of Saint Mark*, c. 1630

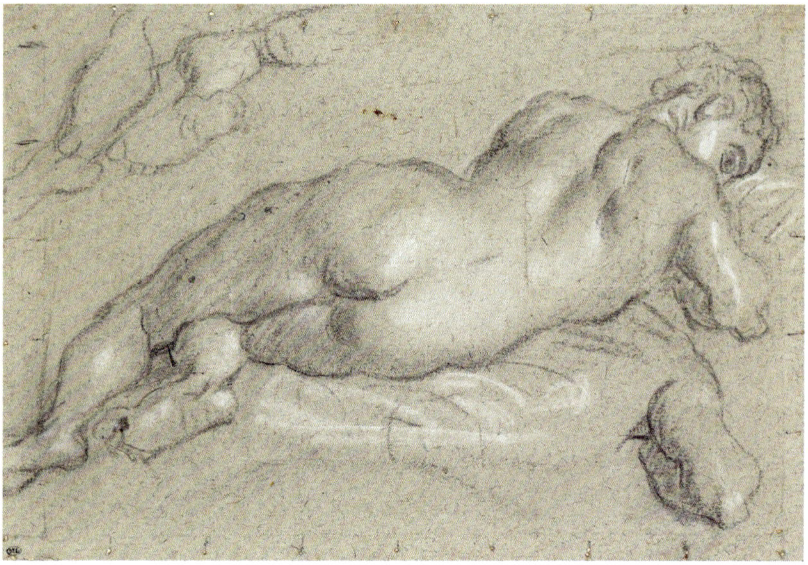

FIG. 16

the Carracci's reform, Domenico uses these sketches to turn Jacopo's aesthetic on its head: nature, with all its flaws, is intentionally given preference over art.

In parallel to these studies from life, Domenico produced a large number of sketches in mixed media on paper. At the outset, these studies acted as a support for the creative process, allowing the painter to clarify the compositional structure of the work and investigate its narrative balance.[20] Eventually, they became definitive works in their own right, whose expressive potential Domenico took to extremes.[21]

An example of the first case is the sketch for the *Miracle of the Ring of Saint Mark* (cat. 11), perhaps made in the 1590s in preparation for the large canvas in the Scuola Grande di San Marco (cat. 4).[22] The drawing documents an advanced stage in the elaboration of the image, in which the painter is investigating the effects of light on the bodies of the members of the confraternity, already clearly distributed within the space of the picture. Completely different, however, is the case of the figure at the center of the composition, the scene's protagonist.[23] The figure stands out for the absence of clothing, which shows that Domenico was still studying the representation of its anatomy. Deft strokes of black paint delineate the rear profile of the body, lending depth to the structure of the ribcage, the tightening of the abdomen, and the reemergence of the hips. In parallel, white lead is skillfully used to emphasize the impact of illumination on the figure's arm and chest, while the reappearance of the dark ground alongside the body lends substance to the taut muscles of the back. The result is a figure with an extremely sculptural modeling that Domenico must have

FIG. 16
DOMENICO TINTORETTO, *Reclining Female Nude and Other Studies*, recto, c. 1580, Paris, Musée du Louvre

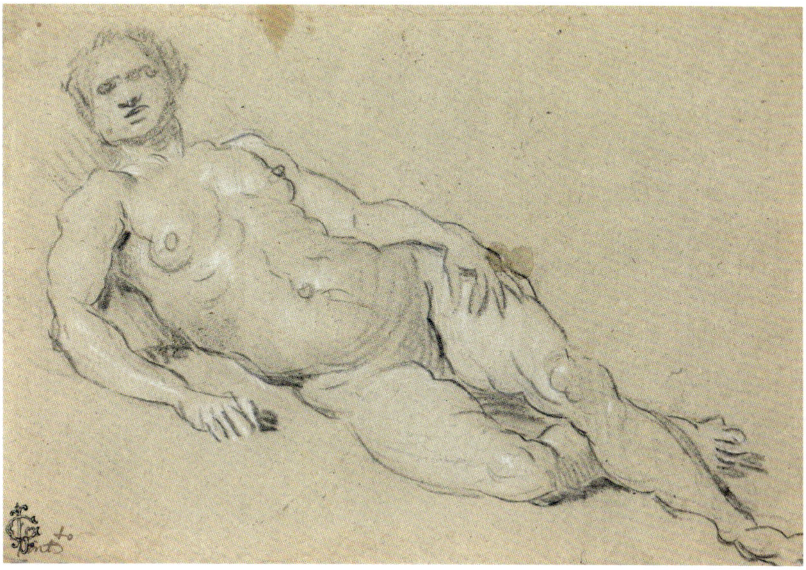

FIG. 17

studied during one or more sessions of drawing from life. In support of this hypothesis we propose a comparison with the folio in the Morgan Library that has already been cited more than once, where the male figure on the left displays numerous affinities of pose and musculature. Put together, these two drawings clarify the outcome of copying Michelangelo's statues, which, in the practice of the workshop, had to be assimilated and become part of the formal baggage of each of its trainees.

As time passed, Domenico's sketches turned into a means of inner meditation, indications of a dialogue the painter held in his own mind in which the reworking of his father's prototypes mirrored a phase of restless research. It is in this production that the rejection of the workshop's style reaches a new expressive peak. One example, out of many, is provided by the five variants of Jacopo's *Miracle of the Slave* for the Scuola Grande di San Marco (c. 1548), produced by Domenico in preparation for the canvas of the same name for the church of Santi Marco e Andrea on Murano (c. 1615–25).[24] The scene, which is brightly lit and carefully measured in Jacopo's version (fig. 4), becomes dark and congested in Domenico's (British Museum, London, 1907,0717.23-27). Figures in leaden colors crowd around the body of the slave, transformed into grotesque masks in whose features we see an echo of the model whose mannishness had already undermined traditional aesthetic canons. Yet it is the depiction of the slave that diverges most from his father's prototype; the flesh tones, previously pure and unsullied, are broken down in Domenico's version into unnatural shades, producing a figure whose physical torment mirrors that of his soul.

FIG. 17
DOMENICO TINTORETTO, *Study of a Female Nude*, c. 1590–1600. Paris, Fondation Custodia, Collection Frits Lugt

An extreme example of Domenico's aesthetic reform is his study in oil on paper for the votive painting *Venice Supplicating the Virgin to Intercede with Christ to End the Plague,* now in the Princeton University Art Museum (cat. 7, fig. 13).[25] This piece may have been produced during the most troubled period in Domenico's life as, facing the potentially fatal effects of the plague for the second time, he was made fully aware of the precariousness of human existence. Although inverted with respect to the final canvas, the study presents an already clearly structured composition which focuses almost exclusively on the personification of Venice as it begs for divine intervention. The sole, glaring exception is represented by a group of plague victims, whom Domenico chose to pile up in the foreground: involuntary and defenseless witnesses to the collapse of life in the city. For some time now the poses of the corpses have been compared with the sketches in the Metropolitan,[26] where, as already mentioned, Domenico brought the ideal beauty of a *Sleeping Venus* into the sphere of the real. In this study, the artist's questioning of the sixteenth-century ideal of beauty appears complete at last. In the process of turning away from a mythical and ahistorical beauty, Domenico first elevated the imperfection of the human body to the status of an aesthetic canon, and then he emphasized its ineluctable transience by depicting the rotting flesh of plague victims. At the age of seventy, Domenico had broken away definitively from the artistic tradition to which Jacopo had made him the sole heir.

With the exception of family members and pupils, it is hard to tell who and how many of Domenico's contemporaries actually had access to his drawings. However, there may be something to Ridolfi's hypothesis that the "disgust" the elderly Domenico felt for the painters of his time stemmed in part from their indifference, if not downright aversion, to an aesthetic that was too radical to be understood, and certainly too distant from the theories on drawing that friends (Palma il Giovane) and colleagues (Odoardo Fialetti and Giacomo Franco) were publishing in those years (cat. 59).[27] One of these artists must have been Ridolfi himself, whose silence on the subject smacks more of censorship than of indifference. Indeed, it is worth quoting a well-known passage from his biography of Domenico, according to which, for a certain period the artist had considered turning his house into an academy, stocked with "the reliefs, drawings and models of his father that he possessed."[28] Despite his respect for Domenico, Ridolfi believed that the only graphic material he owned that would be of use for the education of painters were those sheets produced by Jacopo, and certainly not the hundreds of drawings his son had made, which he passed over in silence.

Ridolfi's censorship soon had its effects. Just over twenty years later Marco Boschini left Domenico out of his list of artists of the *Sette maniere*: painters worthy "of great esteem" who, unlike Jacopo's successor, had chosen to follow in the worthy footsteps "of Titian, Tintoretto, and Paolo Veronese."[29]

NOTES

1 C. Ridolfi, *Le maraviglie dell'arte*, ed. D.F. von Hadeln (Rome: SOMU, 1965), Vol. 2, 11–77.

2 E. Weddigen, "Ein Blick aus Tintorettos Werkstatt in Venedig," in *Künstlerhäuser von der Renaissance bis zur Gegenwart*, ed. E. Hüttinger (Zurich: Waser Verlag 1985), 61–74.

3 L. Whitaker, "Tintoretto's Drawings after Sculpture," in *The Sculpted Object, 1400-1700*, ed. S. Currie and P. Motture (Aldershot: Scolar Press, 1997), 177–191.

4 Ridolfi 1965, 13–18.

5 Ibid., 257–63.

6 S. Mason, "Domenico Tintoretto e l'eredità della bottega," in *Jacopo Tintoretto. Actas Del Congreso Internacional Jacopo Tintoretto/ Proceedings of the International Symposium* (Madrid, Museo Nacional del Prado, February 26–27 2009), ed. M. Falomir (Madrid: Museo Nacional del Prado, 2009), 84–90.

7 C. Ridolfi 1965, 257. For an antithetical interpretation to the one proposed here, see T.M. Zarrillo, "The Neurosis of Visual Legacy: Seicento Venetian Painters Confront Their Past," in *The Enduring Legacy of Venetian Renaissance Art*, ed. A. Badiee Banta (London, New York: Routledge, 2016), 11–24.

8 C. Whistler, *Venice & Drawing 1500-1800. Theory, Practice and Collecting* (New Haven, London: Yale University Press, 2016), 129–45.

9 R. Krischel, "Tintoretto religioso," in *Tintoretto*, ed. G. Morello and V. Sgarbi (Milan: Skira, 2012), 53–54, exhibition catalogue.

10 P. Rossi, "Jacopo Tintoretto: disegni respinti, precisazioni attributive," *Arte Veneta*, 64 (2007), 86, 99–100, nos. 49–50.

11 Ibid., "Disegni della bottega di Jacopo Tintoretto," *Arte Veneta*, 68 (2011), 64, 75.

12 Ibid.

13 S. Mason (ed.), *Palma il Giovane, 1548-1628. Disegni e dipinti* (Milan: Electa, 1990), exhibition catalogue (Venice, Museo Correr, January 20-April 29 1990).

14 Rossi 2007, 60–62.

15 Whistler 2016, 138.

16 G. Feigenbaum, "Practice in the Carracci Academy," in *The Artist's Workshop*, ed. P.M. Lukehart (Washington, DC: National Gallery of Art, 1993), 59–76.

17 P. Rossi, "Per la grafica di Domenico Tintoretto. II," *Arte Veneta*, 38 (1984), 57–71.

18 Ridolfi 1965, 13, 18.

19 A. Forlani Tempesti, *The Robert Lehman Collection. V. Italian Fifteenth- to Seventeenth-Century Drawings* (New York: Metropolitan Museum of Art/Princeton: Princeton University Press, 1991), 136–47.

20 M. Koshikawa, "I disegni di Domenico Tintoretto. Un contributo," *Arte Veneta*, 48 (1996), 56–69.

21 L. Freeman Bauer, "'Quanto si disegna si dipinge ancora'": Some Observations on the Development of the Oil Sketch," *Storia dell'Arte*, 32 (1978), 45–57; R. Rearick, *Il disegno veneziano del Cinquecento* (Milan: Electa, 2001), 205–07.

22 P. Rossi, "Per la grafica di Domenico Tintoretto," *Arte Veneta*, 29 (1975), 205–211.

23 G. Matino, "Per una nuova lettura dell'*Apparitio* di Domenico Tintoretto: il *Miraculum de anulo beati Marci*," in *La Scuola Grande di San Marco a Venezia*, 2 Vols., ed. G. Ortalli and S. Settis (Modena: Franco Cosimo Panini, 2017), 161–64, 270–71 no. 265.

24 P. Rossi, "Temi marciani di Domenico Tintoretto," *Arte Veneta*, 59 (2002), 246–51.

25 See Gear, this volume.

26 Ibid.; Forlani Tempesti 1991, 138.

27 See Klestinec, this volume.

28 Ridolfi, *Le maraviglie...*, 262–63.

29 M. Boschini, "Breve Instruzione," foreword to *Le ricche Minere della Pittura Veneziana* (Venice: Francesco Nicolini, 1674), c. d6.

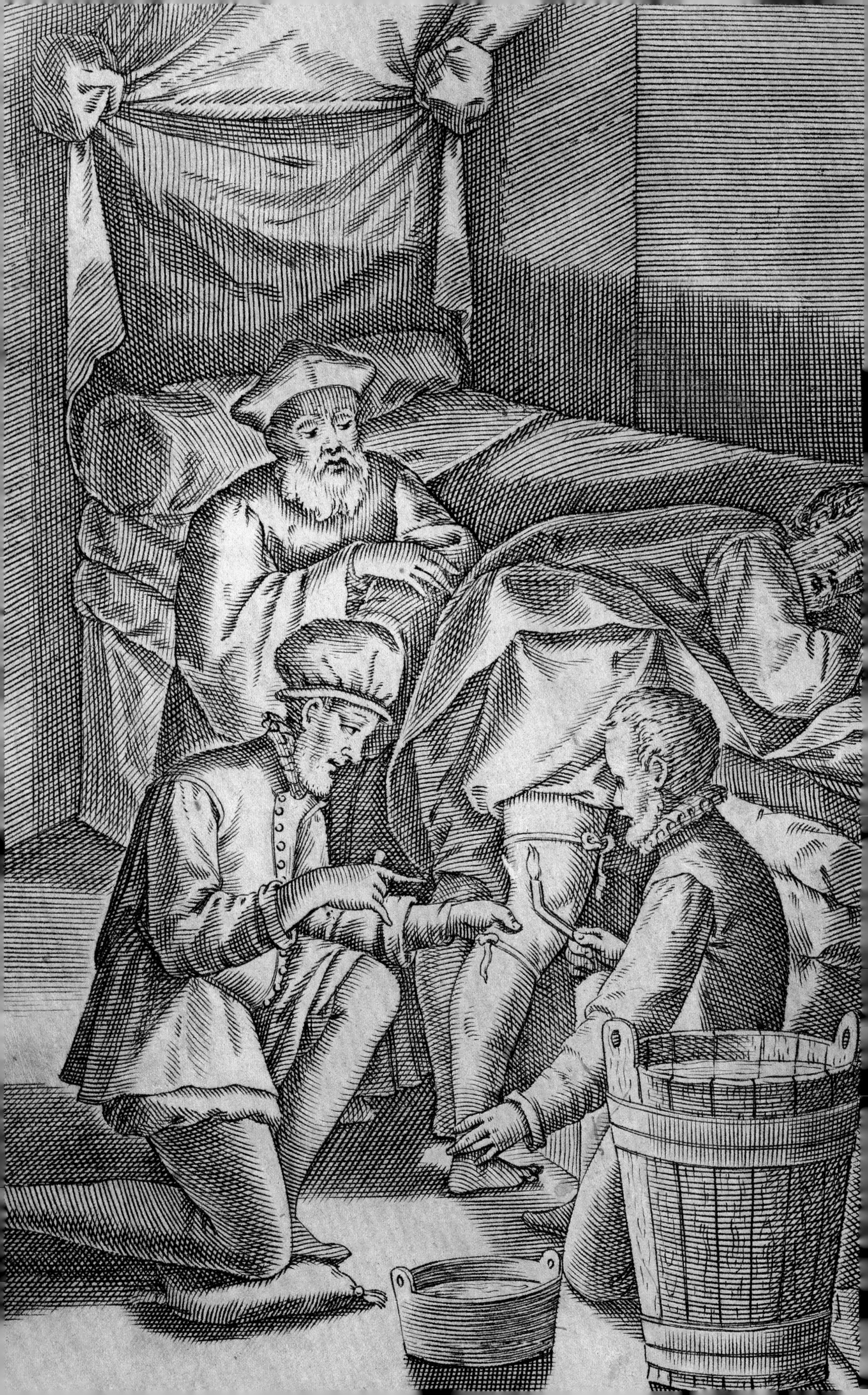

LEARNED HANDS: SKILLS, EXPERIENCE, AND KNOWLEDGE IN SIXTEENTH-CENTURY SURGERY

Paola Savoia

WHEN SCIPIONE MERCURIO (c. 1550–1615) — a student of medicine in Padua and Bologna, a Dominican friar, and a medical practitioner — faced the variety of practitioners who called themselves, and were called by others, "surgeons," he had to address a few puzzling issues. In his *De gli errori popolari d'Italia libri sette* (1603), he acknowledged the confusion of categories between different kinds of surgeons and, almost like a sociologist of health care professions, he attempted an explanation. Mercurio asked why so many people used to put their trust and lives in the hands of such "ignorants" as barbers, wise women, and all sorts of "empirics," that is, people who were not trained in medical schools but who apprenticed with other empiric surgeons.

In Padua — Mercurio claimed — one could not treat surgical illnesses unless one was licensed by the College of Physicians. The problem was that "these men, when they get a license, they think they have a doctorate too, and so believe the people, who begin to call them Doctors, and they [the licensed surgeons] are so charmed by this kind of language that they believe the people." Furthermore, the common people were confused by the fact that they saw "that some Doctors of Medicine practice surgery, and for this reason they are called Surgeons." This is why the empirics could become persuaded, and tried to persuade the public, that they were surgeons just like the surgeons who had graduated from university medical schools.[1]

Moreover, "all Doctors of Medicine are doctors of surgery, and no simple surgeon can be a Doctor too."[2] Here, Mercurio tried to explain why there were graduate physicians who practiced surgical procedures. As he indicates, not all graduate physicians practiced surgery, only those "licensed manual operators" who "have the guts" and who were therefore "allowed to treat wounds and abscesses, clean rotten parts, and apply bandages and plasters." Mercurio sensed that there was much at stake for a graduate in medicine who decided to practice surgery in sixteenth-century Italy: not only was this graduate faced with a wide range of procedures, but also with the possibility of attracting wealthy patrons, and the chance to work in a highly innovative area of medicine.

Let us take a step back. The status of surgery in the Renaissance and in the multifaceted medical tradition known as Galenism has always been clear in theory, but not so clear in practice. In Galen's humoralist system, medicine was divided into three branches: physic, pharmacy, and surgery. Galen and his followers emphasized the unity of the three parts, which together made up the entire edifice of medicine. Physic concerned the inner parts of the

FIG. 18
PIETRO PAOLO MAGNI, *Discorsi di Pietro Paolo Magni piacentino sopra il modo di sanguinare, attacar le sanguisughe, & le ventose, far le fregagioni & vessicatorij a corpi humani*, Rome, Bartolomeo Bonfadino nel Pellegrino, 1586. Venice, Biblioteca di Storia della Medicina del Polo Culturale e Museale Scuola Grande di San Marco

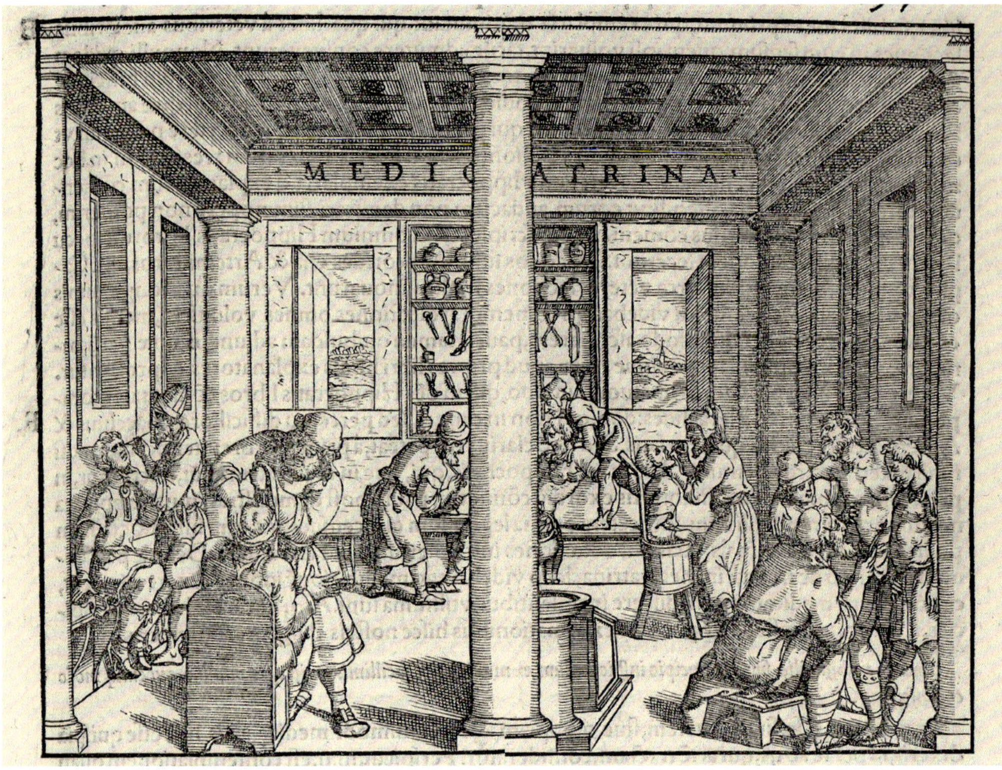

CAT. 44

human body, the invisible ones. From a therapeutic point of view, physicians were those who were able to prescribe oral medicaments — compounds of herbs and animal substances, but also food and drink (diet). Apothecaries were those who had the practical skills necessary to concoct medicaments and handle medical substances, but they were intellectually dependent on the physicians. Finally, surgeons were those who dealt with ailments or diseases which concerned the external parts of the body: all kinds of swellings and skin diseases, but also wounds, fractures, eye conditions, tooth conditions, hernias, stones, and the like (cat. 44).

Though surgeons had to use their hands in their practice, and though they mostly dealt with solid organs and the mechanics of bodily functions, surgical conditions in the Galenic system were commonly defined as "diseases." These could come both from within the body (ulcers, tumors, etc.) and from outside it (wounds, etc.). Moreover, causes were assigned to all surgical conditions, and these causes ultimately led back to humoral imbalances or corruptions. Specifically, surgical diseases were believed to be caused either by a dissolution of continuity (wounds and fractures) or by humoral imbalances (ulcers and tumors).[3]

CAT. 44
CLAUDIUS GALENUS, *Galeni Septima classis. Curandi methodum...*, Venice, 1550

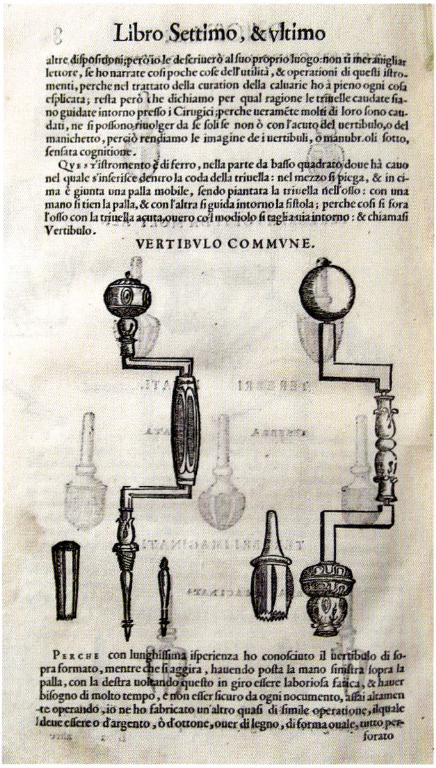

Libro Settimo, & vltimo

altre dispositioni; però io le descriuerò al suo proprio luogo: non ti merauigliar lettore, se ho narrate cosi poche cose dell'utilità, & operationi di questi istromenti, perche nel trattato della curation della caluarie ho à pieno ogni cosa esplicata; resta però che dichiamo per qual ragione le triuelle caudate siano guidate intorno presso i Cirugici; perche ueramēte molti di loro sono caudati, ne si possono riuolger da se soli se non ò con l'acuto del uertibulo, o del manichetto, perciò rendiamo le imagine de i uertibuli, ò manubr.oli sotto, sensata cognitione.

QVEST'istromento è di ferro, nella parte da basso quadrato doue hà cauo nel quale s'inserisce dentro la coda della triuella: nel mezzo si piega, & in cima è giunta una palla mobile, sendo piantata la triuella nell'osso: con una mano si tien la palla, & con l'altra si guida intorno la fistola; perche cosi si fora l'osso con la triuella acuta, ouero co'l modiolo si taglia uia intorno: & chiamasi Vertibulo.

VERTIBVLO COMMVNE.

PERCHE con lunghissima isperienza ho conosciuto il uertibulo di sopra formato, mentre che si aggira, hauendo posta la mano sinistra sopra la palla, con la destra uoltando questo in giro essere laboriosa fatica, & hauer bisogno di molto tempo, e non esser sicuro da ogni nocumento, assai altamente operando, io ne ho fabricato un'altro quasi di simile operatione, ilquale deue essere o d'argento, ò d'ottone, ouer di legno, di forma ouale, tutto perforato

CAT. 49

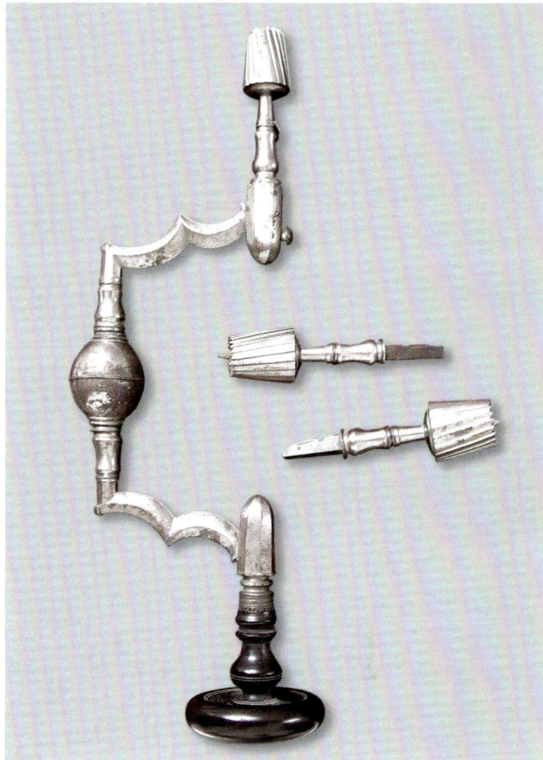

CAT. 73

Italy occupied a special place in the landscape of Renaissance surgery. Indeed, surgery had become an academic specialty in Italian universities by the late thirteenth century. This tradition of academic surgery continued to develop steadily up till the sixteenth century; among other things, it constituted the foundation for the period's famous studies of anatomy, conducted by anatomists who were in fact professors of surgery. This was not the case in most northern European countries, where surgery was mostly an "empiric" enterprise, practiced by people who did not have academic training.

Historians of early modern societies have emphasized the fact that the study of surgeons is still in its infancy.[4] Indeed, one of the most puzzling features of early modern surgery is that the title of surgeon seems to describe very different kinds of practitioners: from barbers to bonesetters, from those hired by the city to treat the people for free to university-trained physicians, from hernia specialists to peddlers of unguents and potions.

CAT. 49
GIOVANNI ANDREA DALLA CROCE, *Cirugia vniuersale e perfetta di tutte le parti pertinenti all'ottimo chirurgo*, Venice, 1583

CAT. 73
Cranium drill and bits, second half of the sixteenth century

In European cities the typical sixteenth-century institutional arrangement could take three forms. The first was a division between a College of Physicians, a College of Surgeons whose members were also scholars, and a guild of barber-surgeons. Examples of this arrangement could be found in Venice and some northern cities. In the second type of arrangement, learned surgeons belonged to the College of Physicians, while surgical practitioners who lacked a university degree belonged to the barbers' guild or were independently licensed by the College. This arrangement could be found in Bologna and Padua. The third type of arrangement, which was more widespread north of the Alps, consisted in a distinction between a guild of barber-surgeons and a College of Physicians: here, surgeons shared their practice with barbers and were excluded from the College of Physicians.[5]

The Colleges of Medicine, whose members were elite physicians who had graduated from universities, greatly expanded their functions. Almost everywhere on the Italian peninsula, Colleges were placed side by side with the Protomedicati, medical magistracies charged with policing the boundaries among health care providers and medical practitioners. Italian Protomedicati and Colleges of Physicians tried to enforce the threefold partition of the medical professions with greater and lesser degrees of success.[6] Colleges and Protomedicati were not professional associations, but an aristocracy, a self-affirming ruling medical elite. Their aim was not to ban all illicit practice, but to affirm their right to rule and be recognized as the top of the medical hierarchy.[7] Colleges acknowledged the existence of three kinds of surgeons: those with an academic degree in surgery; physicians who chose or wanted to practice surgery; and people with no academic degree but with a certified path of apprenticeship with a master surgeon.

During the sixteenth century, the Colleges extended their jurisdiction to barber-surgeons, a crucial category of practitioners. Indeed, barber-surgeons were tasked both with cutting hair and beards, and performing important surgical tasks, particularly bloodletting or phlebotomy. Bloodletting was the most common form of both preventative and therapeutic medical intervention in Renaissance Europe. It consisted of cutting one of the patient's veins so that noxious humors may seep out along with the blood. It was performed with lancets, cupping glasses, and leeches. It was supposed to heal fevers and pains, evacuate bad humors (from the body as a whole, but particularly from the stomach), and even calm the patient's nerves.

Bloodletting had both a scholarly and a practical/technical pedigree. All classical Greek and Arabic authorities, including Hippocrates, Galen, and Ibn-Sina (Avicenna) had written about it. However, by the late Middle Ages, its practice had been entrusted to barbers and empirically trained surgeons. As a result, by the second half of the sixteenth century, barber-surgeons began to write books about their trade (fig. 18). Along with an abundance of technical details about how to skilfully use their hands and tools, they also began to take pride in their profession, and to cast light on its important history.

The scholarly physician accepted this development, but cast himself in the role of supervisor. The Colleges and the Protomedicati could grant licenses to practitioners who specialized in single procedures, such as the extraction of

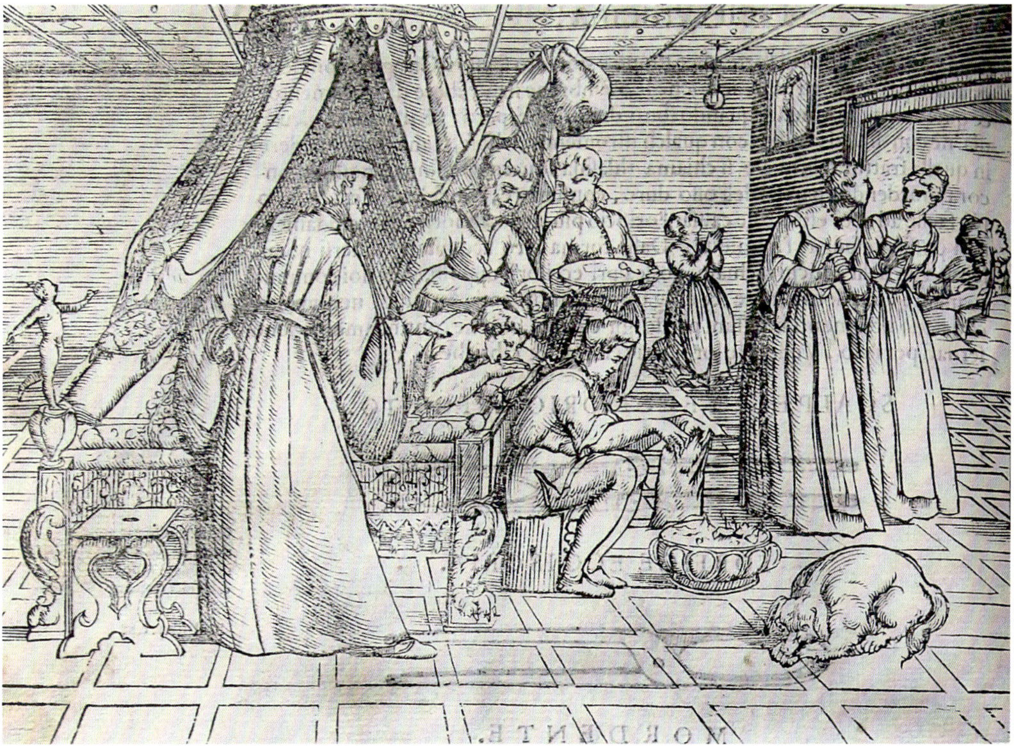

CAT. 49

hernias and stones (in the case of Norcia's so-called *norcini*), the treatment of cataracts, dentistry, etc.[8]

Just as barber-surgeons had begun to cast light on the important history of their practice, educated surgeons began to describe in new, more robust ways all aspects of their profession. Nearly all Renaissance surgery books, regardless of whether they were written in Latin or in the vernacular, included a description of the "ideal" learned surgeons. Usually such descriptions combined elements that had remained constant from the times of Celsus and Galen. They defined the moral, technical, and cognitive qualities of surgeons. In particular, Celsus's definition of the ideal surgeon, together with a passage from the Hippocratic corpus recommending the dexterity of the practitioners' hands,[9] formed the standard picture that medieval and Renaissance learned surgeons always reiterated. Celsus's surgeon had to be "youthful or at any rate nearer youth than age; with a strong and steady hand which never trembles;" he had to have "sharp and clear sight." As for his moral qualities, which constituted a kind of complement to his scientific equipment, the good surgeon's "spirit" had to be "undaunted"; he must be "filled with pity, so that he wishes to cure his patient, yet is not moved by his cries, to go too fast, or cut less than is necessary; but he does everything just as if the cries of pain cause him no

CAT. 49
GIOVANNI ANDREA DALLA CROCE, *Cirugia vniuersale e perfetta di tutte le parti pertinenti all'ottimo chirurgo*, Venice, 1583

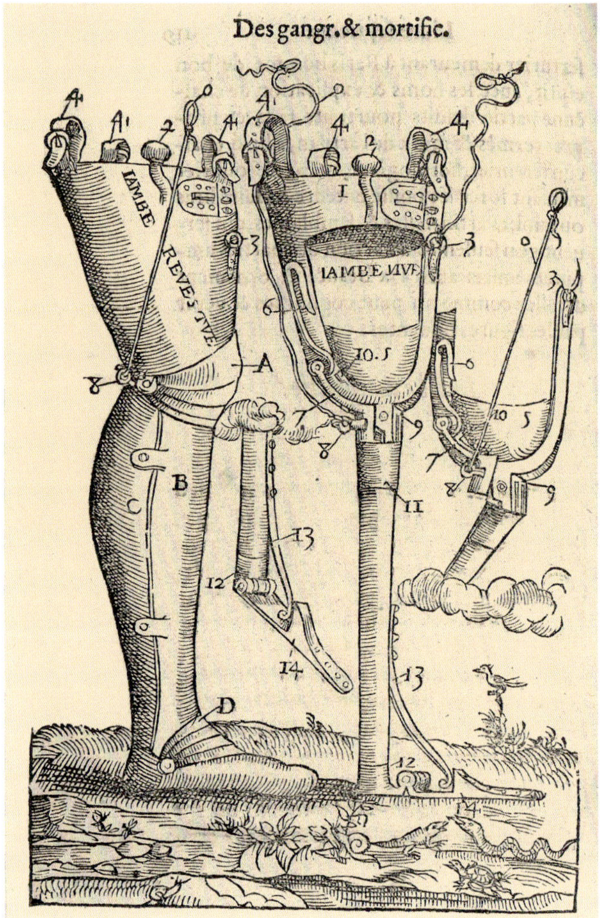

CAT. 50

emotion."[10] Sixteenth-century surgeons' definitions combined more or less the same elements, but placed more emphasis on technological innovation and the surgeons' abilities to minimize pain. The Venetian Giovanni Andrea dalla Croce describes an ideal surgeon who can also be an "inventor of new instruments" and "ready to promise to restore the patients' health"[11] (cat. 49, 73). Another typical theme in sixteenth-century descriptions of the ideal surgeon is the "learned hand,"[12] a phrase that emphasized the intertwining of theory and practice, manual skill and medical education. Finally, even educated surgeons did not disdain comparisons with artisanship and the world of crafts; surgeons could learn how to stitch and measure skin from tailors, how to stop the blood flow from executioners, how to design instruments from engineers, and how to bandage damaged limbs from farmers.[13]

CAT. 50
AMBROISE PARÉ,
Opera chirurgica...,
Frankfurt, 1594

But what was surgery for a sixteenth-century practitioner? Giovanni Andrea dalla Croce defines surgery as "operationi delle mani," and he adds that "this is the most difficult and tiring of the parts of medicine, but also the most ancient and noble, and more certain than the other parts, that which treats many illnesses with the hands and several instruments." Croce defines surgery as "an ability of the practical intellect, that can be acquired through many rules and experiments, aiming at healing quickly and with small pain through artful operations of the hand and the proper instruments, by joining, separating, and taking away many diseases in the continuum of the parts of the body." This manual operation is made with "order, art, and prudence, and not without a certain grace; it is ruled by anatomy and by extensive practical experience [*una lunga prattica*]." Its goal is "restoring the unity of the body's parts." Surgery is based upon the most accurate knowledge of anatomy, but it is very different from anatomical operations, in that it operates on living bodies, not on dead ones (cat. 49).[14]

This scholarly conception should not to be taken as the norm at the time. For example, the empiric surgeon Leonardo Fioravanti was highly skeptical of the work of learned surgeons, and he often rhetorically exalted the natural remedies one could learn from the wisdom of nature, as opposed to the complex, painful, and technologically advanced procedures of university-trained surgeons. Fioravanti bitterly criticized the practice of skull trephination, which was used to treat fractures, as too "artificial." He wrote that he could not understand how physicians could possibly justify treating skull fractures by cutting and dilating the bones of the head. "But above all I marvel," he added, "at how the wounded patients let themselves be tortured for no plausible reason."[15] Fioravanti advocated patient non-compliance: he believed that patients should rebel against the pain educated surgeons needlessly inflicted on them. Instead of the learned surgeons' agonizing, destructive procedures, Fioravanti believed that skull wounds should be treated with the application of ointments and other external remedies that he concocted and sold himself. Elsewhere, he went so far as to question the value of anatomical studies for surgeons:

> Instead of learning so much anatomy, we would do better to learn agriculture, to treat surgical conditions more easily and in a simpler manner, without tormenting the patient ... because for patients it is much better to have the right remedies than to let their wound be observed in detail: for this reason, the former [the caring surgeon] comforts and the latter [the anatomically-skilled educated surgeon] tortures; the former heals, the latter kills.[16]

In the sixteenth century, the word "surgery" referred to a complex and broad array of practices, institutions, and people. Sixteenth-century surgeons were also aware that surgery granted more room for innovation and experimentation than other branches of medicine. The Bolognese learned surgeon Gaspare Tagliacozzi devoted an entire monograph to a very difficult skin-grafting operation, intended to restore lost or mutilated parts of the face, especially noses.[17] By the sixteenth century, particularly in northern Europe, surgeons, gunsmiths, and clockmakers had begun to design and assemble mechanical limbs, thus creating emotional and technical bridges between human and non-human objects (cat. 50).[18] The empirically trained barber-surgeon Ambroise Paré, who became the most important practitioner of the century, was able to build on his experiences of treating gunshot wounds directly on the battlefield, and come up with a new method for treating this new kind of injury. While serving as a war surgeon in Piedmont in 1536, Paré had only read about such wounds in Giovanni da Vigo's authoritative handbook. Da Vigo claimed that there was poison in the wounds, because of the poisonous nature of gunpowder, and thus recommended that the surgeon cauterize such wounds with oil of elder, theriac (a famous medical recipe) or — a more practical suggestion — boiling oil. One day, short of oil, Paré simply applied oil of roses, eggs, and turpentine to the wound he was treating. Fearing that the patient would die of poison, the morning after Paré rushed at his bedside, only to find that he was "feeling very little pain, with neither inflammation nor tumor." After repeating the procedure with several other patients, always successfully, Paré concluded: "From then I resolved never again so cruelly to burn poor men wounded with arquebus shot."[19]

NOTES

1 S. Mercurio, *De gli errori popolari d'Italia libri sette* (Padua: Francesco Bolzetta, 1645), book 3, 208.

2 Ibid., 209: "Ogni Dottor di Medicina è anco dottor di cirugia, e niun cirugico semplice può essere Dottore."

3 For an overview of the Galenic system, see N. Siraisi, *Medieval and Early Renaissance Medicine* (Chicago, London: University of Chicago Press, 1990).

4 F. de Vivo, *Information and Communication in Venice: Rethinking Early Modern Politics* (Oxford: Oxford University Press, 2007), 101; S. Cavallo, *Artisans of the Body in Early Modern Italy: Identities, Families and Masculinities* (Manchester, New York: Manchester University Press, 2010), 1–7.

5 On the early institutional and academic teaching of surgery in medieval Italian universities see Siraisi 1990, 153–86; T. Pesenti Marangon, "'Professores chirurgie,' 'medici ciroici' e 'barbitonsores' a Padova nell'età di Leonardo Buffi da Bertapaglia († dopo il 1448)," *Quaderni per la Storia dell'Università di Padova* (Journal of the History of the University of Padua) 11 (1978): 1–38; M. McVaugh, *The Rational Surgery of the Middle Ages* (Florence: SISMEL/Edizioni del Galluzzo, 2006). On early modern surgery, see R. Palmer, "Physicians and Surgeons in Sixteenth-Century Venice," *Medical History*, 23, 4 (1979): 451–60; D. Giordano, "Venezia ne' suoi chirurghi: il Collegio iatro-chirurgico," in ibid., *Scritti e discorsi pertinenti alla storia della medicina e ad argomenti diversi* (1930), 59–93; D. Gentilcore, *Medical Charlatanism in Early Modern Italy* (Oxford: Oxford University Press, 2006), 182–87; M. Conforti, "Chirurghi, mammane, ciarlatani. Pratica medica e controllo delle professioni," in *Il Rinascimento italiano e l'Europa. Volume 5: Le scienze*, ed. A. Clericuzio and G. Ernst (Treviso: Angelo Colla Editore, 2008), 323–340.

6 D. Gentilcore, "'All That Pertains to Medicine': Protomedici and Protomedicati in Early Modern Italy," *Medical History* 38, 2 (1994): 121–42.

7 G. Pomata, *Contracting a Cure: Patients, Healers, and the Law in Early Modern Bologna*, trans. the Author, R. Foy, and A. Taraboletti-Segre (Baltimore: Johns Hopkins University Press, 1998).

8 D. Bartolini, "On the Borders: Surgeons and their Activities in the Venetian State (1540-1640)," *Medical History*, 59, 1 (2015): 83–100.

9 G. Cosmacini, *La vita nelle mani. Storia della chirurgia* (Rome, Bari: Laterza, 2003), 27.

10 Celsus, *De medicina*, 3 Vol., trans. W. G. Spencer (Cambridge: Harvard University Press, 1935–38), Vol. 3, 297.

11 G.A. dalla Croce, *Cirugia universale e perfetta* (Venice: Giordano Ziletti, 1583), 6r-6v.

12 See T. Garzoni, *La piazza universale di tutte le professioni del mondo*, 2 Vols., ed. P. Cherchi and B. Collina (Torino: Einaudi, 1996), Vol. 1, 207.

13 See, respectively, C. D'Amato, *Prattica nuova et utilissima* (Venice: Giovanni Battista Brigna, 1669), 8; G. Gentili, *La vita e l'opera di Bartolomeo Maggi* (Bologna: Università di Bologna, 1967); C. Klestinec, "Renaissance Surgeons: Anatomy, Manual Skill, and the Visual Arts," in *Early Modern Medicine and Natural Philosophy*, ed. P. Distelzweig, P.B. Goldberg, and E.R. Ragland (Dordrecht: Springer, 2016), 43–58. On surgeons as artisans see Cavallo's groundbreaking *Artisans of the Body* (2010).

14 Dalla Croce 1583, 1r-2r.

15 L. Fioravanti, *La Cirurgia* (Venice: 1570), Vol. 2, 119v.

16 Ibid., 119r, 143v.

17 P. Savoia, "Nature or Artifice? Grafting in Early Modern Surgery and Agronomy," *Journal of the History of Medicine and Allied Sciences*, 72, 1 (2017): 67–86.

18 J. Gagné, "Emotional Attachments: Prosthetic Iron Hands, their Makers, and their Wearers, 1450-1600," in *Feeling Things: Objects and Emotions through History*, ed. S. Holloway, S. Downes, and S. Randles (Oxford: Oxford University Press, 2018), 133–53.

19 A. Paré, *Oeuvres completes*, 3 Vols., ed. J.-F. Malgaigne (Paris, Baillière, 1840), book 8, 126–27. Translation by I.M.L. Donaldson, from ibid., "Ambroise Paré's Accounts of New Methods for Treating Gunshot Wounds and Burns," *Journal of the Royal Society of Medicine* 108, 11 (2015): 457–61.

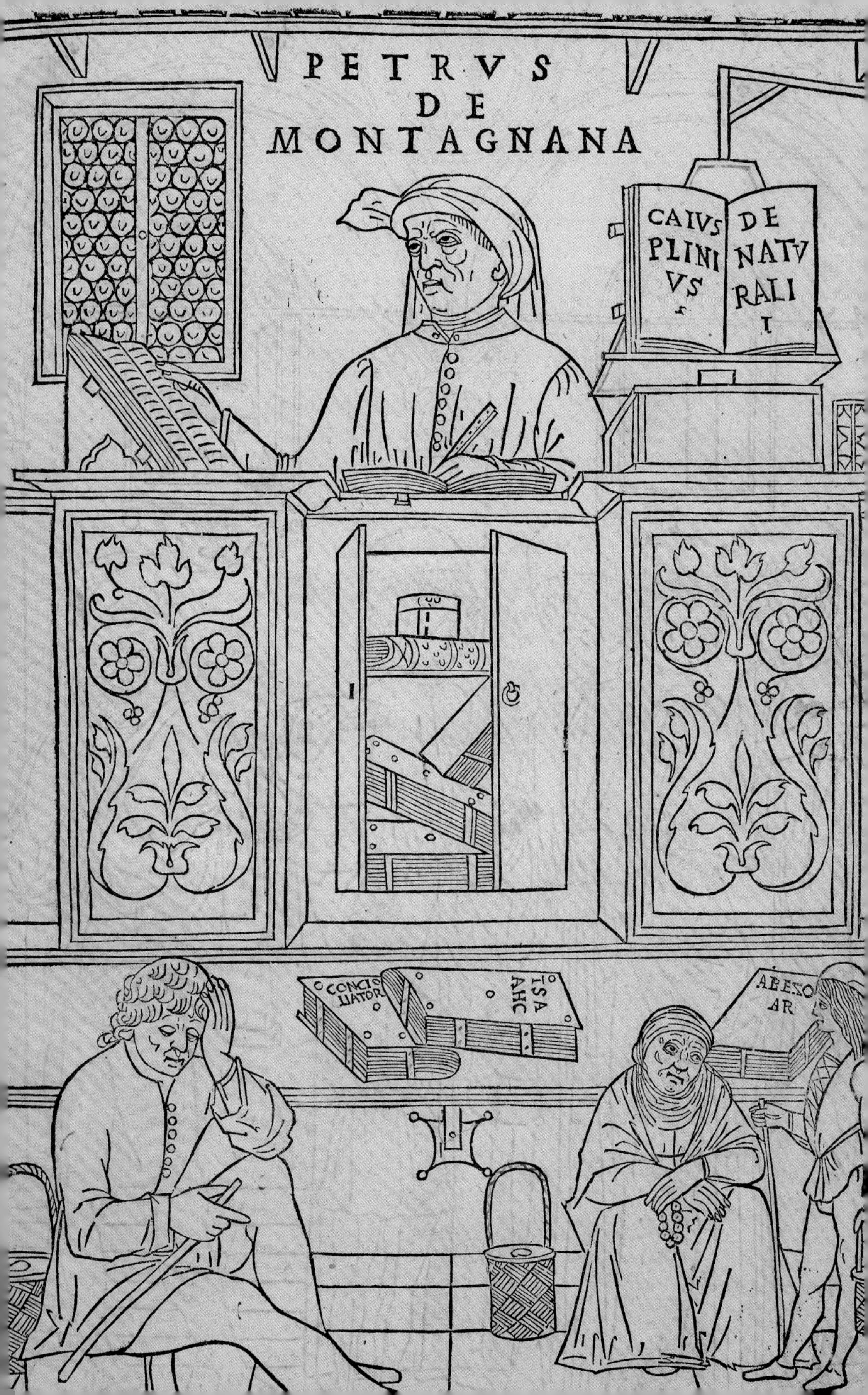
PETRVS
DE
MONTAGNANA
CAIVS PLINIVS
DE NATVRALI
CONCI LIATOR
ISA AHC
ABEZO AR

BOOKISH ANATOMIES: THE MEDICAL MANUAL IN THE FIRST CENTURY OF PRINTING

Ilaria Andreoli

IN THE SECOND HALF of the fifteenth century, movable-type printing combined the novelty of mass production with traditional kinds of content and formal characteristics associated with the manuscript. Because room was so often left for accessory and decorative elements, it soon became necessary to decorate the printed page with woodcut or xylographic figuration and ornamentation. This was the main technique used for the illustration of *incunabula* and books published in the sixteenth century.

In a woodcut, the lines of the drawing, made directly on the wood or on a sheet of paper that is then glued onto its surface, are cut into small blocks of fairly soft types of wood (pear, sycamore, or beech); then with a saw, the lines are traced along the grain (unlike in wood engraving), sanded, and left to season to avoid warps or cracks.

Movable metal types and woodblocks were based on the principle of relief printing. That is, they marked paper with protruding parts covered in ink. Metal types and woodblocks had the same thickness of about 2.5 centimeters, and both could be placed in the matrix, together, and then inked and printed on the sheet of paper using the same press.

In the 1480s and 1490s, woodcut illustrations grew increasingly sophisticated, as the marking of just the outlines (known as a white-line woodcut) was gradually replaced by an engraving that could produce chiaroscuro effects and the illusion of volume by means of shading with parallel or cross-hatched lines. As the sixteenth century progressed, the use of the woodcut was usually limited to framings and flourishes, while *intaglio* or copperplate engraving (also known as chalcography), despite its considerably greater cost, slowly came to dominate illustration. This technique, in which the ink fills grooves, had to be printed on a different press and separately from the text. While it permitted finer lines and images of greater complexity and sophistication, it required that illustrations be located on plates separate from the text, marking the end of the union between words and images.

In the sixteenth century, modern typography attained a level of splendid perfection, and its extraordinary development meant that the medical manual flourished too. The conjunction of the rise of the printed book as the principal means of spreading information with the reformulation of the means of visual representation that took place during the Renaissance was an integral part of what we call the Scientific Revolution.[1]

CAT. 52 JOHANNES DE KETHAM, *Incipit fasciculus medicine...*, Venice, 1513

The most popular medical books of the time were the works of Galen and Hippocrates, especially when it at last became possible to read the original and complete versions in Greek or Latin, editions often edited by illustrious physicians as well as contemporary scholars. Then came the other classical authors, especially Oribasius, Dioscorides, and Paul of Aegina, though the Arab writers continued to be published and read as well, always in Greek or Latin translation. Alongside the great masters of antiquity, contemporary specialists in anatomy, surgery, and pharmacopoeia like Berengario da Carpi, Andreas Vesalius, Juan Valverde, Hieronymus Fabricius, Jean Tagault, Giovanni Andrea dalla Croce, and Pietro Andrea Mattioli were proving ever more popular.

Venice was the home of medical publishing since the fifteenth century, with Basel as its sole rival. Venice had become a true center of Greek culture following the fall of Constantinople (1453), thanks to the manuscripts that exiles had been able to save from the latter city's pillage. Although it was not the seat of a university, Venice's printers were able to sell their volumes to the numerous students and professors from nearby Padua, and, above all, they were able to benefit from the immense commercial network that distributed them by land and sea to markets all over Europe. Along with Basel, it was Lyon that had the most important role — on both the national and European scale — in the production of books on medicine, mostly in small formats like octavo, duodecimo, and sextodecimo, which became particularly widespread after 1525, and which were preferred by both professionals and, given their low cost, students. However, for luxury editions of Galen, Hippocrates, and the Greek classics, folio remained the most popular format, and before long anatomists realized that illustrations, which were essential to their studies and work, were more effective on larger plates.

While medical *incunabula* were rarely illustrated, their sixteenth-century editions can certainly be counted among the most beautiful books of the day, due to their figured title pages and abundant engravings, often of notable artistic quality. In the sixteenth century, human figures, which in the previous century had been depicted in poses of hieratic rigidity, started to come to life, and the didactic contribution of the text, especially in the major treatises of anatomy, was complemented by the presence of numerous plates of incontestable artistic value. An increasingly demanding clientele began to expect illustrations that were not just attractive, but, more importantly, also accurate. Besides physicians, they were purchased by people who had nothing to do with medicine except as patients (canons, lawyers, other members of the wealthy bourgeoisie), and who, to satisfy their curiosity and broaden their knowledge, started to take an interest not just in the theoretical bases of the great masters of antiquity, but also in the results of the first steps toward the application of the experimental method based on direct observation. Vesalius's *Fabrica* (1543) not only returned to Galen but also affirmed new ways to study the human body. At the same time, it ushered in a new era

CAT. 42
JOHANNES
DE KETHAM,
Fasciculus medicinae,
Venice, 1491

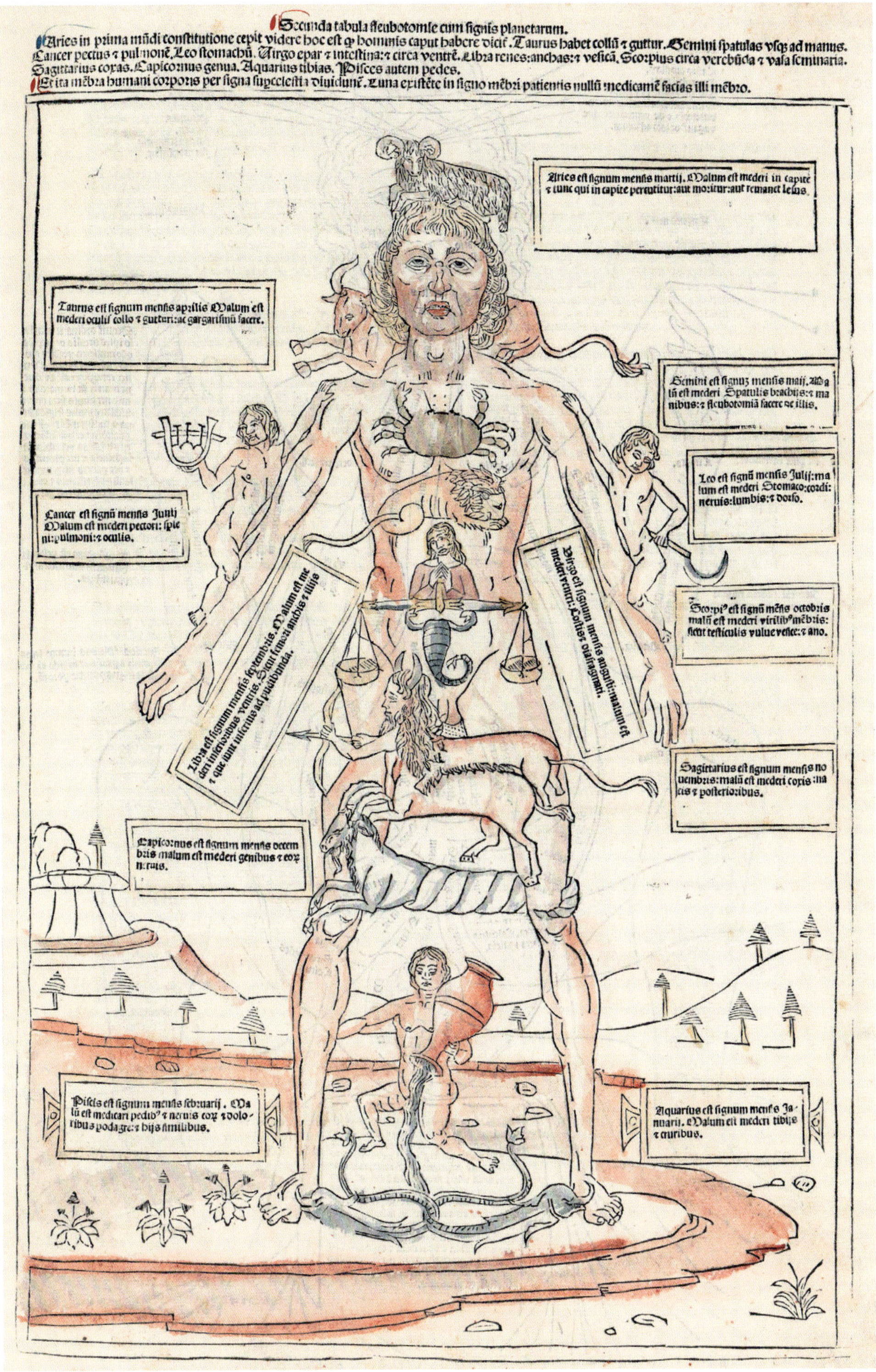
Secunda tabula fleubotomie cum signis planetarum.
Aries in prima mūdi constitutione cepit videre hoc est q̃ hominis caput habere dicit. Taurus habet collū ⁊ guttur. Gemini spatulas vsq̧ ad manus.
Cancer pectus ⁊ pulmonē. Leo stomachū. Virgo epar ⁊ intestina: ⁊ circa ventrē. Libra renes: anchas: ⁊ vesicā. Scorpius circa verēbūda ⁊ vasa seminaria.
Sagittarius coxas. Capicornus genua. Aquarius tibias. Pisces autem pedes.
Et ita mēbra humani corporis per signa supcelestia diuidunt. Luna existēte in signo mēbri patientis nullū medicamē facias illi mēbro.
Aries est signum mensis martij. Malum est mederi in capite ⁊ tunc qui in capite percutitur: aut moritur: aut remanet lesus.
Taurus est signum mensis aprilis Malum est mederi oculis collo ⁊ gutturi: ac gargarismū facere.
Gemini est signū mensis maij. Malū est mederi Spatulis brachijs: ⁊ manibus: ⁊ fleubotomiā facere de illis.
Cancer est signū mensis Junij Malum est mederi pectori: splenis: pulmoni: ⁊ oculis.
Leo est signū mensis Julij: malum est mederi Stomaco: cordi: neruis: lumbis: ⁊ dorso.
Libra est signum mensis septembris. Malum est mederi inferioribus ventris. Sicut femori anchis ⁊ illis ⁊ que sunt inferius ad pudibunda.
Virgo est signum mensis augusti: malum est mederi ventri: Costis: diafragmati.
Scorpi⁹ est signū mēsis octobris malū est mederi virilib⁹ mēbris: sicut testiculis vulue vesice: ⁊ ano.
Sagittarius est signum mensis nouembris: malū est mederi coxis: anchis ⁊ posterioribus.
Capicornus est signum mensis decembris malum est mederi genibus ⁊ cornerus.
Piscis est signum mensis februarij. Malū est medicari pedib⁹ ⁊ neruis eor ⁊ doloribus podagre: ⁊ hijs similibus.
Aquarius est signum mensis Januarij. Malum est mederi tibijs ⁊ cruribus.

CAT. 42

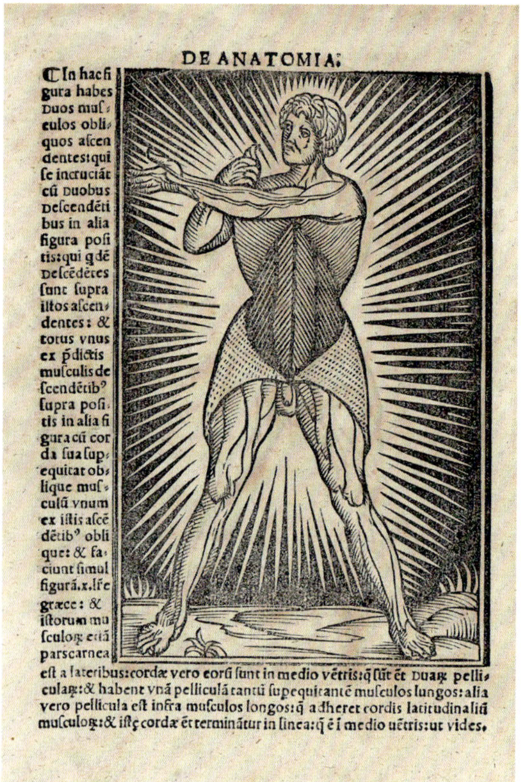

CAT. 35

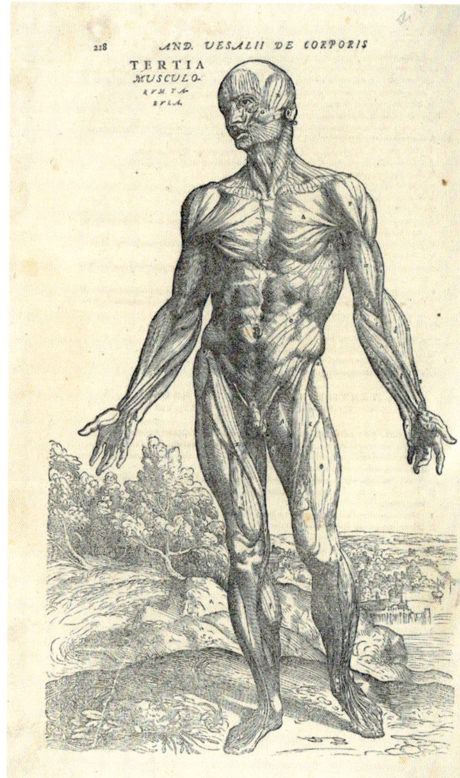

CAT. 38

of anatomical illustration making it an indispensable point of reference for almost two centuries to come.

At the beginning of the sixteenth century, the bases of medical knowledge in the Western world were the *Hippocratic Corpus*, the theory of the four humors (also attributed to Hippocrates), the anatomical teachings of Galen, and the cardiocentrism of Aristotle. Yet the schools of medicine imparted almost exclusively the doctrine of the Arabs, while only a few Latin translations of the great Greek masters existed, which were themselves based on often corrupt and incomplete Arabic versions. The emergence of the *ars artificialiter scribendi*, or the art of writing by mechanical means, whose invention in Germany had coincided with the fall of the Eastern Roman Empire, permitted the rapid spread of the new knowledge throughout Europe. A new generation of humanists and scholars, for whom it was now possible to consult the original sources, began editing, translating, and commenting on the ancient authors. Thus physicians of the sixteenth century were able to read all the great classical writers on medicine, now available in their original texts or in excellent Latin translations.

CAT. 35
JACOPO BERENGARIO DA CARPI, *Anatomia Carpi. Isagoge breues...*, Venice, 1535

CAT. 38
ANDREAS VESALIUS, *Andreae Vesalii Bruxellensis, ... De humani corporis fabrica...*, Basel, 1555

While this rediscovery of antiquity was taking place, anatomy, which until then had been long neglected, began to make great strides. If for artists it underpinned an ever more attentive approach to the accurate representation of the body, for doctors it came to constitute the very heart of a discipline that was increasingly reliant on scientific observation. Moreover, at the time, it became increasingly common for professors to carry out dissections personally instead of presiding over the operation from on high, delegating the task of cutting into the body to an assistant. In addition, certain specific circumstances also favoured the regeneration of the art of surgery. Of these, the most important one was, doubtless, the invention of firearms, as they caused new, deeper wounds that were more difficult to treat, which stimulated a continual search for new treatments. A passion for the observation of nature and reality more widely, combined with a renewed interest in the writings of the ancients, finally led to a more exacting study of plants, including ones introduced as a result of geographical discoveries, which in turn led to new therapies and pharmaceutical remedies.

The earliest book on medicine in which we find the high artistic quality and elegant line of the Renaissance woodcut is the first Italian edition of the *Fasciculus medicinae*, published in 1493–94 in Venice by Giovanni and Antonio de' Gregori, and reprinted several times over the course of the century (cat. 52). Commonly attributed to Johannes de Ketham, this collection of eight late-medieval texts on medical and surgical topics was presented not just as a conceptual summary but also, thanks to its ten woodcuts, as a visual synthesis of medical teaching and practice. Published in Latin in 1491, the work was originally illustrated with six anatomical woodcuts, which were carefully colored by hand. The ten woodcuts in the Italian edition can be divided into two groups. The first, comprising reworkings of the six illustrations of the Latin edition, is made up of descriptive plates, including the *Zodiac Man* (cat. 42), who is surrounded by the twelve signs that govern the different parts of the body and their frailties. The second is made up of four images that were introduced in the first vernacular edition (brought out in 1493–94), and they are very different from the others: lacking captions, they can be regarded as the "mute" title pages of the collection, providing a vivacious account of four moments in the daily life of physicians and their patients — the visit to the doctor, the urine test, the examination of a plague victim, and an anatomy: an illustration that, in many copies, including the one in the exhibition, is colored *à pochoir*, a precursor of the stencil technique (cat. 33).

An early anatomical text to be illustrated in the modern sense of the term is the work of Jacopo Berengario da Carpi. In his *Commentaria* (1521), he built on the lessons of his teacher, the celebrated Bolognese professor Mondino de Luzzi, with twenty-one illustrations whose style was still fairly crude but in which the human body is caught in the dramatic and pathetic poses that from then on would animate bodies and skeletons in print. Despite their undoubted novelty, these illustrations, accompanied by descriptive captions (cat. 35) that give them a relative autonomy of interpretation, performed a strictly limited anatomical function in relation to the text, and, when referring to them, the author does so in terms that restrict their role. More than half of these images were used again in the compendium of anatomy titled *Isagogae breves* that Berengario also published in Bologna the following year. This time, he added several new pictures, though they were again rather schematic, notwithstanding the pathos of the poses representing the internal organs. Thus we come to the middle of the century and to the period of lavishly illustrated treatises.

In 1543, the first edition of the Flemish physician Andreas Vesalius's *De humani corporis fabrica* (cat. 38) was published in Basel, on the presses of Johannes Oporinus.[2] That same year, its *Epitome*, containing nine plates and a summary of the text, also came out, in Latin and German. The title page (cat. 37) is not just a masterpiece of sixteenth-century xylography, but also an extremely complex and remarkably intricate image that the author freighted with numerous meanings, often in close relationship to his text, and whose execution he personally supervised. The same can be said for the other three hundred woodcuts in the book. Probably made in Venice from drawings by Jan Steven van Calcar, a pupil of Titian, and subsequently sent to Basel for printing, they are divided into twenty-five tipped-in plates and a large number of vignettes of various sizes inserted in the text. In them, Vesalius tried out the whole range of illustrations at his disposal — anatomical charts, drawings of dissections, three-dimensional sections, isolated systems, separate and united forms, variable points of view, and a series of diagrammatic concepts — displaying incredible assurance in selecting the most appropriate image for the text to which it refers. Through the annotations to the plates, he conducts an unprecedented dialogue with the reader, in which the visual presentation serves as a surrogate for the experience of an eye witness, or as a visual synthesis of many such experiences. Like all the finest books of the century, the *Fabrica* is also embellished with historiated initials peopled by anatomist and surgeon putti that offer views in miniature of contemporary practices (cat. 38). The excellent typographical quality achieved by Oporinus was one of the reasons for the immediate success of the *Fabrica*, whose plates for over two centuries were to remain an obligatory point of reference for later works that were either inspired by them or, more simply, that copied them outright.

The best-known imitator — and counterfeiter — of Vesalius was the famous Spanish anatomist Juan Valverde de Amusco, whose *Historia de la composicion del cuerpo humano*, a translation of Vesalius's text with some alterations, was published in Rome in 1556. Some of the forty-two copperplate engravings, made after drawings by Gaspare Becerra (known for having worked with Michelangelo on the Sistine Chapel), are inverted with respect to their models, while others appear to have been modified. Only two of them are new, including a flayed figure inspired by Michelangelo's depiction of Saint Bartholomew in the *Last Judgment* (cat. 39). Although it permitted a greater refinement in the details, the

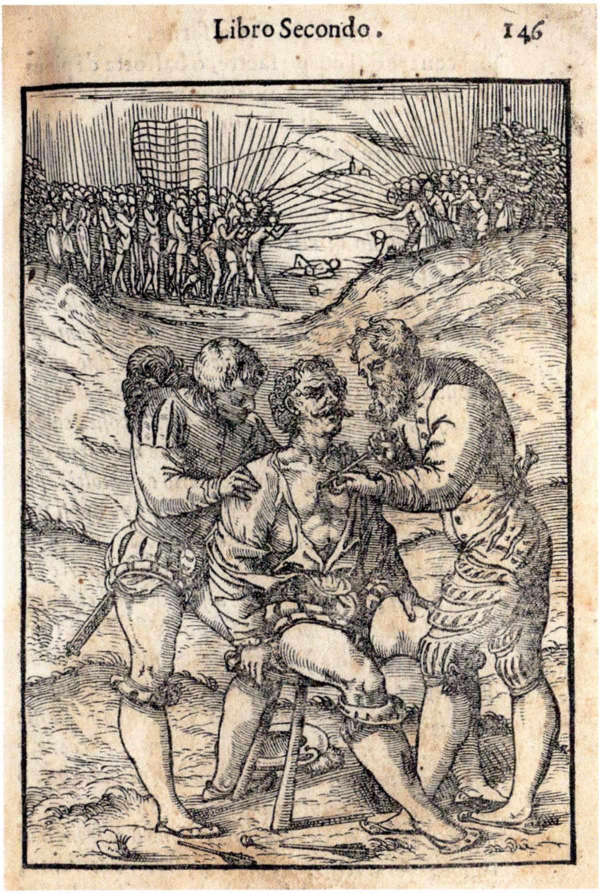

CAT. 51

choice of copperplate engraving caused some difficulties in the organization and printing of the plates. They were all included in the Italian translation of the work, whose *editio princeps* came out in Rome in 1560.

However, the influence of Vesalius was not solely limited to the major treatises that had so faithfully reproduced the plates of the *Fabrica*, nor did it cease at the end of the century. Indeed, it is worth mentioning the anatomical treatises of Iulius Caesar Casserius and Hieronymus Fabricius (cat. 10), published at the turn of the sixteenth century. The former devoted himself chiefly to the study of anatomical parts governing the five senses, making comparisons between the human and the animal. Fabricius (Casserius's teacher) also followed a more comparative approach, and he was the author of numerous monographic works on individual disciplines that made significant contributions to anatomy, physiology, and embryology, all of them illustrated with large copperplate engravings.

CAT. 51
JEAN TAGAULT,
De chirurgica institutione,
Venice, 1596

48 A *Pro modiolo etiam poteris lecto mediocrem trabeculam subijcere, eiusq; utrunque caput stabilire, lignisque recuruatis lora extendere.*

A Trabecula.
B Ligna recuruata.
C Lora.

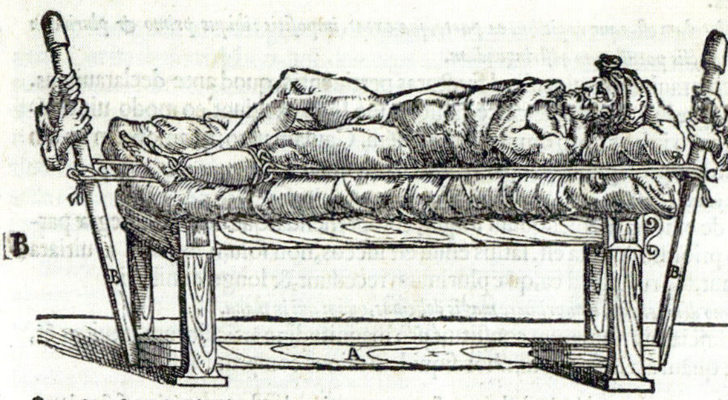

Ante, binis modiolis, binisq; uectibus in contrarias partes extédebat, uno infra pedem extéto, altero supra caput. Sed quoniã (ut retuli) in eo exerceri nos uoluit, ut præsidia in promptu habeamus, aliũ modũ docens, in similiũ inuétione te exercet. nã, si modioli non sint, tignum, quod lecti, super quo ægrotans iacet, longitudinẽ æquet, subijciendũ est. Cetera omnia, eadẽ atq; ante efficiẽda sunt. lora enim corpori inijcienda eo modo, quo superius docuit, uinciendaq; ad ligna, quibus, quasi uectibus ad extendendum utimur. Sed pro modiolis nunc adhibentur extrema longioris tigni, quæ capita dicuntur, ut modice utrinq; lectum excedentia, & a capite, & a pedibus, extendẽtibus lignis, mora sint. trabeculam uero, quod lignum in longitudinem lecto subijcitur, δοκίδα dixit, quasi paruam trabem significans.

49 *Commode item extendes per axiculos ab utraque parte collocatos. sunt et aliæ extendendi rationes, quàm plurimæ.*

C

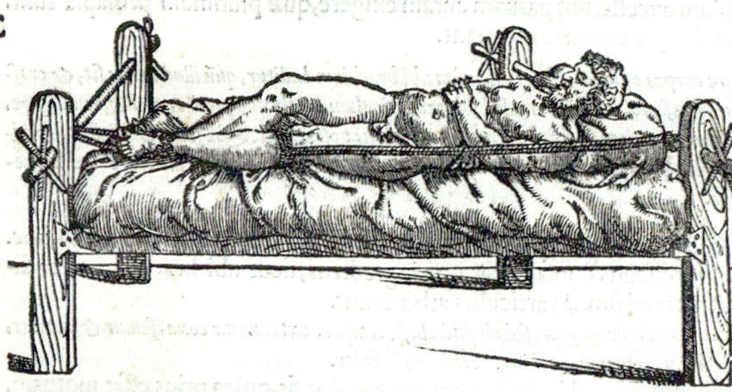

Axes solitus est appellare asellos, quẽadmodũ ubi scribit, Axis uersatio, nunc uero axiculos nominauit ὀνίσκους, usus nomine diminutiuo, sicut in superioribus uerbis, trabeculã dixit, paruam trabẽ significans. Exerceri autẽ debes, non solũ in ijs, quæ própta sunt, excogitandis atq; admouẽdis, sed ẽt in machinamẽtis, quæ parant a medicis ad has intendẽdi rõnes. Axes itaq; collocãdi sunt, nó recti in lõgitudinẽ corporis, sed transuersi ab ijs, quæ hinc, atque hinc sunt, partibus corporis, quod curatur. id autem non aliud significat, quàm alterum ab inferiori parte a pedibus, alterũ a superiori a capite collocandum esse. Post hæc inie-
D cta lora extrema ad axes danda, qui uersati crus, quod curatur, in diuersas partes diducant.

50 *Optimum aũt est, si quis medicinam in magna urbe exerceat, paratum habere lignum, per quod uim omnẽ adhibeamus, ad fracta & luxata omnia restituenda, tum extendentes, tum impellentes. abunde autem erit lignum tale, quales sunt quadratæ columnæ quernæ, quod ad longitudinem, latitudinem, & crassitudinem pertinet.*

Organi cuiusdam, seu machinamenti, quod haberi uoluit, mentionem facit: in libro autem de articulis, qui huic subijcitur, docet eius fabricationem. nos ibi si quid obscurum fuerit, exponemus. nunc proximum est ad ea transire, quæ subdit.

51 *Vbi satis extenderis.*

Crus uidelicet, de crure enim agens circa talum prolapso inseruit extendendi rationem: sicque rursus ad sermonem reuertitur, quem initio proposuit.

52 *Articulus facile reconditur. diducitur enim ab antiqua sede, sic, ut e regione supra ipsam spectans non hæreat. prominentioribus itaque palmarum partibus dirigendus est, partim, quod extat adurgentibus, partim infra talum repellentibus. Eo restituto crus, si fieri potest, extentum alligandum est: sin lora prohibeant, ea soluenda, & dum uinculum inijcitur, in contrarias partes extendendum.*

Hippocrates articulum dixit, quo mouentur, qui uolunt sic apud ipsum uocari extrema ossa, quæ in cauis recipiuntur, sic, ut totum id appelletur articulatio, ubi committuntur extrema ossium, quæ in

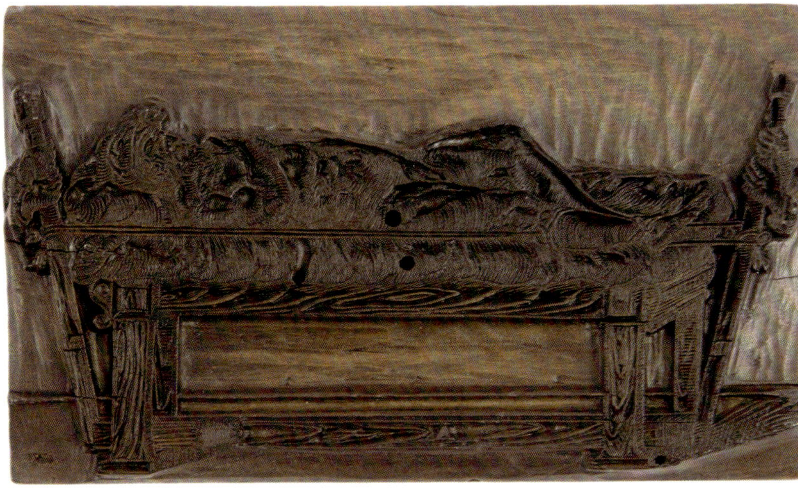

CAT. 63

With few exceptions, sixteenth-century treatises on surgery were not as sumptuous as contemporary anatomy treatises. Usually, they were small octavo volumes, cheap and easy to handle. Indeed, because they were of common use, they have now become quite rare. Their fairly simple and schematic illustrations depicted operating instruments and techniques, and it was not until the end of the century that some authors began to show interest in the quality of the plates to be inserted in their editions.

The best-known name of the early part of the century is that of Giovanni da Vigo, physician to Pope Julius II, whose *Pratica in arte chirurgica copiosa*, published for the first time in Venice in 1514, was followed by a large number of new editions and translations over the entire course of the sixteenth century.

However, it is necessary to wait until the middle of the century to see the appearance in Paris of three large editions that attest to the renascence of surgical studies. Jean Tagault's *De chirurgica institutione*, printed in 1543 and adorned with just five woodcuts and a few drawings of surgical instruments, was republished repeatedly and translated several times (cat. 51). A year later, the Florentine physician Guido Guidi (also known as Vidus Vidius) published his *Chirurgia e graeco in latinum conversa*. This was a collection of texts by various authors, accompanied by Guidi's comments and by numerous illustrations reproducing the fine drawings in pen and bister that Francesco Salviati and his assistants had made (based on the illuminations of a Byzantine codex) on two manuscripts, in Greek and Latin, of the *Chirurgia* to be sent as a gift to the king of France. From these woodcuts were later made other sets of illustrations that accompanied various reissues of the same texts, often included in the *Opera Omnia* of Galen that was printed several times by the Giunti family and by Valgrisi in 1563–64 (cat. 45): miraculously,

CAT. 45
CLAUDIUS GALENUS, *Galeni Omnia, quae extant singulari studio...*, Venice, 1562

CAT. 63
Scene of an anatomical manipulation, wooden block, mid-sixteenth century

seven of this edition's original matrices have survived (cat. 63).[3] In 1575 the complete work of Ambroise Paré appeared, decorated with 295 woodcuts. The illustrations of anatomy were still derived — wholly, in part, or reduced in size — from those of Vesalius, while the surgical ones depicted numerous instruments and even models of artificial limbs. The century closed with a Venetian edition, Giovanni Andrea Dalla Croce's illustrated treatise, which would prove extremely popular right through the seventeenth century.

In the sixteenth-century, studies of the natural sciences, botany in particular, also went through a genuine Renaissance. Specifically, a shift took place from the knowledge of the classical and medieval eras, which focused almost exclusively on identifying the medical properties of plants, to an altered study which was chiefly interested in the description and cataloguing of species. This was partly due to increasingly frequent voyages of exploration, and the subsequent discovery of new systems of flora and fauna, resulting in a wholly new figurative output aimed at a representation of nature that was as realistic as possible. Botanical and zoological treatises included lavish sets of illustrations that provided a useful supplement to the written text, even taking its place on occasion. The main inspiration for this trend, which began in the fifteenth century with the publication of the *Hortus sanitatis*, was the rediscovery of Dioscorides, whose *De Materia Medica*, which had already been published in Latin and Greek versions at the end of the fifteenth century, was reissued several times over the whole of the sixteenth, inspiring many commentators. The most famous of these was undoubtedly Mattioli, who wrote a Latin version of his *Commentaries* for an international readership, and one in Italian for apothecaries with no knowledge of Latin. Both editions were illustrated with hundreds of extraordinary woodcuts depicting animals and plants and based on drawings by Giorgio Liberale.[4]

During the first century of printing, medical books experienced large-scale distribution and commercialization. With lavish sets of illustrations, these books combined traditional and novel forms of inquiry with an imagination that was curious about every aspect of nature, and expressed in a few notable cases, genuine artistic ambitions. Later, following the adoption of copperplate printing, and as a consequence of a doctrinal turn in the discipline, medical books would move, in their text as well as in their illustrations, toward increasingly academic styles and forms.

NOTES

1 A. Carlino, *La fabbrica del corpo. Libri e dissezione nel Rinascimento* (Turin: Einaudi, 1994); I. Andreoli, "L'invenzione del corpo. Il libro di medicina nel Cinquecento: forme, evoluzione, illustrazione," in *Saperi e meraviglie. Tradizione e nuove scienze nella 'libraria' del medico genovese Demetrio Canevari*, ed. L. Malfatto and E. Ferro (Genoa: Sagep, 2004), 83–128, exhibition catalogue (Genoa, Civica Biblioteca Berio, October 28 2004-January 31 2005); S. Kusukawa, *Picturing the Book of Nature: Image, Text, and Argument in Sixteenth-Century Human Anatomy and Medical Botany* (Chicago: University of Chicago Press, 2012).

2 S. Kusukawa, http://cudl.lib.cam.ac.uk/view/PR-CCF-00046-00036/1

3 I. Andreoli, "Macchine nel tempo. Sette matrici xilografiche, quattro manoscritti e cinque edizioni a stampa illustrati del corpus galenico," *L'illustrazione*, I (2017), 29–48.

4 *I discorsi di P.A. Mattioli. L'esemplare dipinto da Gherardo Cibo: eccellenza di arte e scienza del Cinquecento*, 2 Vols., facsimile and comments (Sansepolcro: Aboca, 2015), 69–85.

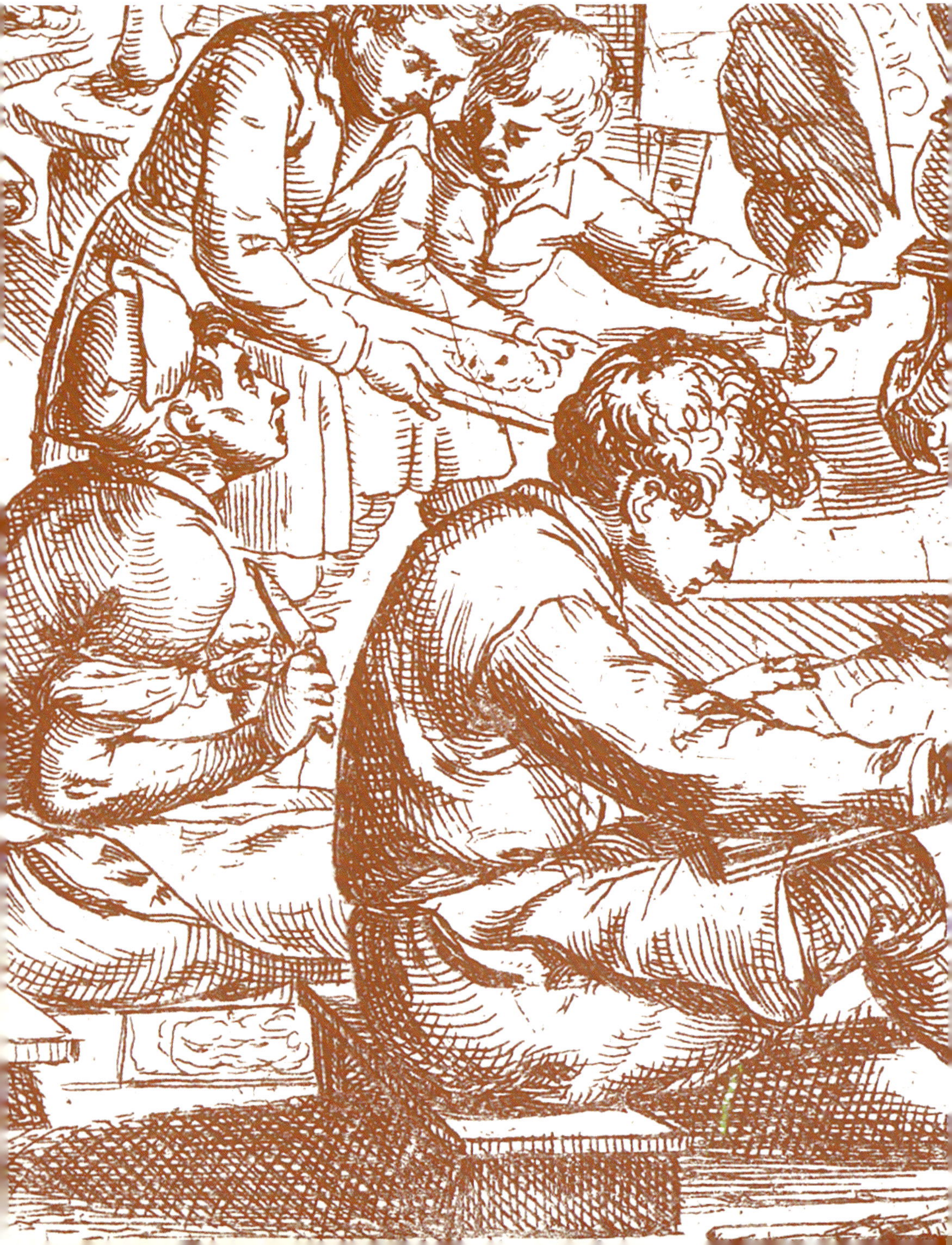

APPENDIX

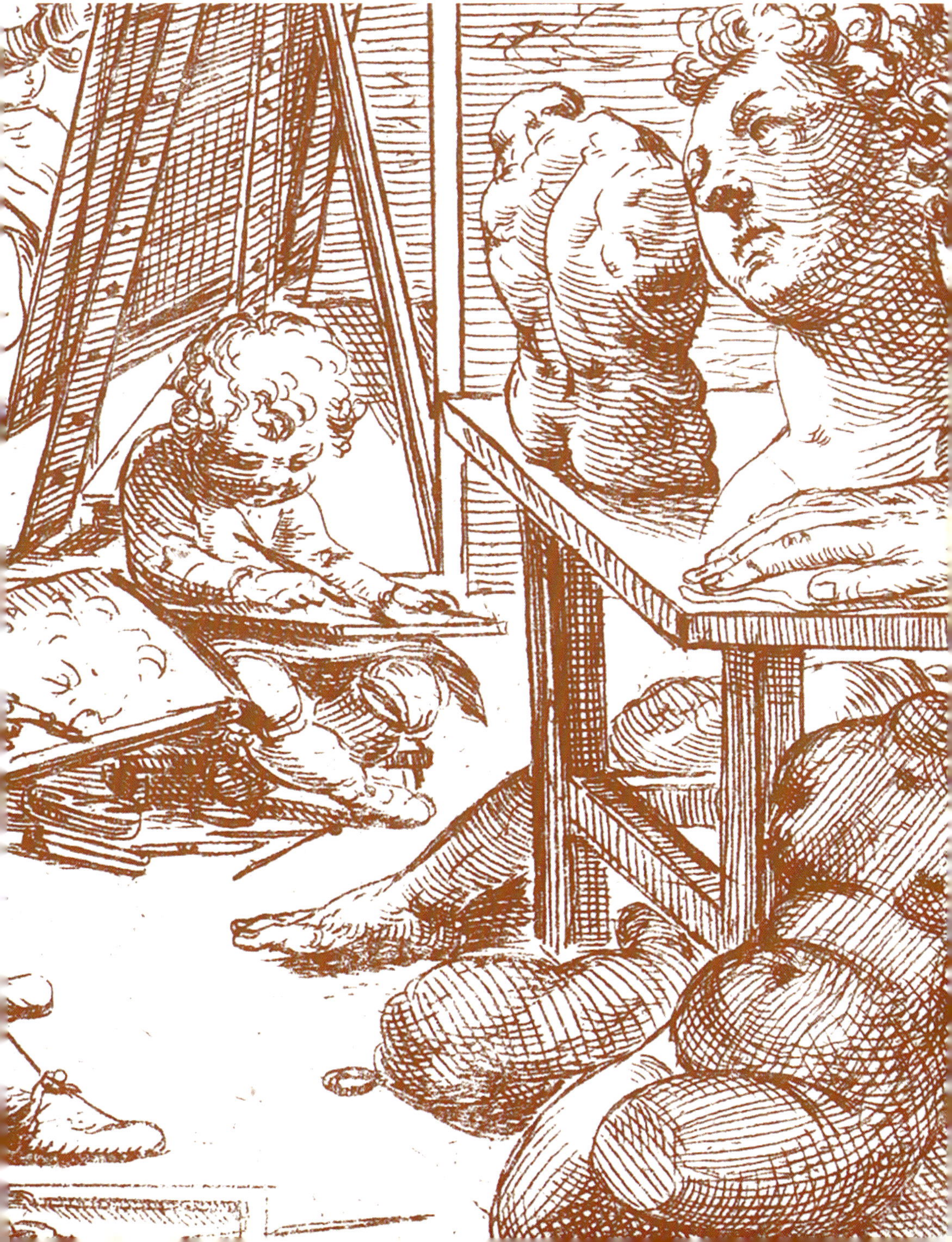

CHRONOLOGY

Gabriele Matino

THE DOCUMENTS RECORDING the activity of Jacopo and Domenico Tintoretto at the Scuola Grande di San Marco have been published at different times, chiefly as a consequence of the fragmentation of research that has characterized study of the subject. A first corpus of documents was compiled thanks to the pioneering work of Pietro Paoletti (1929). These were then supplemented by scholars focusing on the history of the Scuola's architecture (Sohm 1982) or on the biographies of distinguished members of the confraternity (Weddigen 1978) and those of the painters who worked on its decoration (Moschini 1965–66; Krischel 1991; Mancini 2017; Sclosa 2017). Reorganized and arranged in chronological order, these documents allow us to examine the cycles of canvases painted by Jacopo and Domenico in the light of wider questions. A first useful insight is provided by their involvement in the activities of the confraternity. As brethren more than painters, Tintoretto father and son were integrated into the social fabric of the Scuola, exploiting the opportunities it offered in much the same way as all the artists who had preceded them — including, among others, Gentile and Giovanni Bellini. Documents suggest that Jacopo obtained the initial commission for the decoration of the Chapter Hall in part thanks to his ability to take advantage of ties of kinship and relations of patronage established with the Scuola's elite. The same circumstance emerges from documentation regarding Domenico, who was able to rely on his connections with the Scuola's officials or *banca*, and was therefore able to continue his father's work until the balance of power shifted away from him, but not without first putting up a fight with the help of the faction that remained favorable to him. Many avenues for future research remain, above all with regard to the officials, and the oligarchic groups they belonged to, who played key roles: by promoting the cycle of paintings, holding competitions, selecting artists, instructing them with regards to the content of their work, and sometimes rejecting the results and even hindering a work's conclusion. Together these officials and their activities comprised a campaign of decoration that lasted for over half a century.

NOTE

For reasons of concision, almost all the documents have been paraphrased. The only exception is the inventory of the "Quadri di Pitture nella Sala Grande" (1681), which has been transcribed in full, as it records the position of the canvases in the rooms of the Scuola and, as such, is the basis for the remounting of the cycle of paintings in the chapel presented in this exhibition. References to the archives and to the modern publication in which it is possible to find a transcription in full of the document cited, or in which it was made known for the first time, may be found in the margin of each entry. Owing to gaps in the documentation relating to the delivery of Jacopo Tintoretto's four canvases, some contemporary literary sources are cited alongside the papers in the archives.

I would like to express my gratitude to Doctor Paola Benussi and Doctor Giovanni Caniato of the State Archives of Venice for having facilitated the activity of research, consultation, and transcription of the documents.

ABBREVIATIONS

ASVe	*Archivio di Stato di Venezia*
SGSM	*Scuola Grande di San Marco*
c.	*carta* (sheet)
fasc.	*fascicolo* (file)
reg.	*registro* (register)
b.	*busta* (file)
r.	*recto*
v.	*verso*

1542
November 30 – The Guardian Grande and Soprastante alla Fabbrica (Superintendent of Construction) Stefano Buontempo orders the start of work on the decoration of the Sala Capitolare with paintings that will depict "scenes from the life of our patron Messer [Master] Saint Mark."

ASVe, *SGSM*, reg. 19 (Notatorio 1537–45), c. 79r; R. Krischel, *Jacopo Tintoretto 'Sklavenwunder'* (Munich, 1991), 197–99

1544
October 28 – During a session of the *banca* chaired by Gasparo Bevilacqua, the canvases Stefano Buontempo had commissioned are criticized, having been "authorized by him without speaking to anyone," and the *banca* votes to *reconzar* (improve) them. The name of the artist (or artists) responsible for the paintings is not recorded.

ASVe, *SGSM*, reg. 19 (Notatorio 1537–45), c. 145r; P. Sohm, *La Scuola Grande di San Marco, 1437–1550: The Architecture of a Venetian Lay Confraternity* (New York, London 1982), 289–90 no. 112

1548
January 20 – Jacopo Tintoretto receives "14 lire [and] 8 soldi" from the Guardian da Matin Marco Episcopi, his future father-in-law, for having painted twelve wooden *ferallj da asta* (lamps or lanterns) carved by "Daniel tornidor" (Daniel the turner) vermilion red.

ASVe, *SGSM*, reg. 229 (Libri antichi di contabilità, 1480–1560), fasc. 8; Krischel 1991, 204

1548
April – In a letter sent to Jacopo Tintoretto, Pietro Aretino congratulated him "on the public praise" which had been showered on the "great picture of the scene dedicated in the Scuola" to the *Miracle of the Slave*, at this date already installed on the southern wall of the Sala Capitolare.

Pietro Aretino, *Edizione Nazionale delle opere di Pietro Aretino IV: Lettere*, ed. P. Procaccioli (Rome: Salerno Editrice, 2000), no. 429, 266

1552
June 12 – Owing to the failure to respect the resolution of October 28, 1544, the Guardian Grande Antonio Pellegrini and the Soprastanti alla Fabbrica (Gaspare Bevilacqua, Tommaso Zonta and Giovanbattista Alban) renewed the order to "reorganize, improve, and change everything necessary in the canvases" that Stefano Buontempo had commissioned.

ASVe, *SGSM*, reg. 20 (Notatorio 1545–52), cc. 166–67; Sohm 1982, 293–94 no. 121

1560
April 28 – The Guardian da Matin Costantino da Riva records the payment of the sum of "6 l[ire] 6 s[oldi]" to "Jacomo depenttor" (the painter Jacopo) for painting thirty-six *arme* (coats of arms) on the *ombrelle* of the Scuola.

ASVe, *SGSM*, reg. 229 (Libri antichi di contabilità 1480–1560), fasc. 9; Krischel 1991, 210

1561
December 23 – The Guardian Grande Vittore Garbignan enjoins "the painter Andrea Medola," known as Schiavone, to deliver "the picture that you are obliged to give me by the middle of the next month of Zenaro [January]." The subject of the work was to be the *Apparition of Saint Mark*.

ASVe, *Notarile*, *Atti*, Marino Renio, 11631, cc. 89r–89v; V. Mancini, "Andrea Schiavone e la Scuola Grande di San Marco: qualche riflessione sulla tarda attività," *Saggi e memorie di storia dell'arte*, 38 (2014), 29–32

1562
June 21 – The Guardian Grande Tommaso Rangone decides to "have painted entirely at his expense three pictures with the miracles of our most holy patron Messer Saint Mark," and to decorate the spaces between the windows of the west wall of the Sala Capitolare with "the seven deadly sins and with the seven lasting or opposite [theological and cardinal] virtues." In the same resolution the space "near the Chapel" is reserved for the canvas commissioned by Vittore Garbignan from Schiavone. The work will never be delivered.

ASVe, *SGSM*, reg. 22 (Notatorio 1562–79), c. 4r; E. Weddigen, "Thomas Philologus Ravennas," *Saggi e memorie di storia dell'arte*, 9 (1974), 7–76

1566
May 19–25 – During his stay in Venice, Giorgio Vasari has an opportunity to see, in the Sala Capitolare of the Scuola, in addition to the *Miracle of the Slave*, Jacopo Tintoretto's three canvases depicting, respectively, "a tempest of the sea, and Saint Mark, likewise in the air, delivering another of his votaries," "a storm of rain with the dead body of another of Saint Mark's votaries, and his soul ascending into Heaven," and "an evil spirit [being] exorcised, [in which Tintoretto] counterfeited in perspective a great loggia, and at the end of it a fire that illumines it with many reflections."

G. Vasari, *Lives of the Painters, Sculptors and Architects*, trans. G. de Vere (London: Everyman's Library, 1996), Vol. 2, 513.

1568
May 2 – Jacopo Tintoretto signs a contract with the Guardian Grande Tommaso Rangone to paint, in gouache or oil, the scene of "how the body of Messer Saint Mark was brought to Vinetia [Venice]," for which he was paid eighty ducats.

ASVe, *SGSM*, reg. 22 (Notatorio 1562–79), c. 137r; Weddigen, "Thomas Philologus...," 60

1573
August 10 – The three paintings commissioned from Jacopo Tintoretto by Tommaso Rangone for the Sala Capitolare are removed and sent to the latter's home, but "he did not want them and they were returned to the Scuola."

ASVe, *SGSM*, reg. 22 (Notatorio 1562–79), c. 203r; Weddigen 1974, 60–61

1573
September 8 – The three paintings are transferred to the "house of Messer Jacopo Tentoretto" (sic) so that they can be completed "perfectly by removing the figure of His Excellence Ravenna [Tommaso Rangone]." To this was added the request to finish a "fourth picture of the said Sala [Capitolare], free of charge and out of courtesy."

ASVe, *SGSM*, reg. 22 (Notatorio 1562–79), c. 205r; P. Paoletti, *La Scuola Grande di San Marco* (Venice, 1929), 182

1575
March 11 – The Council of Ten "declares and protests" to the officials of the Scuola, "both present ones and their successors," that the pictures in the Scuola cannot be removed "or anything changed in them" without the prior approval of the Chapter General.

ASVe, *SGSM*, reg. 22 (Notatorio 1562–1579), c. 230v; Krischel 1991, 211

1585
December 28 – Jacopo Tintoretto agrees with the Guardian Grande Pietro Verucci to paint the "pictures and altarpiece" of the Scuola's chapel in exchange for admission to the confraternity, "free of charge and without any expense," of his son-in-law Marco Augusta (husband of Marietta Robusti), his son Giovanni Battista Robusti, the tailor Bartolomeo di Lorenzo, and Angelo Girardi.

ASVe, *SGSM*, reg. 23 (Notatorio 1579–88), c. 158r; Paoletti 1929, 184–86

1586
March 17 – Domenico Robusti is elected *Degano tutto l'anno* (junior member of the *banca*) of the Scuola.

ASVe, *SGSM*, reg. 6 bis (Registro cariche 1440–1743), c. 34v; *SGSM*, reg. 23 (Notatorio 1579–88), c. 167

1586
December 14 – With reference to the resolution of December 28, 1585, the Guardian Grande Luca di Giovan Alvise and the Sindaci (provosts, including Perazzo Perazzi) request "Messer Giacomo Robusti painter and member of our confraternity" to paint the canvases for the chapel. In response to Jacopo's complaint that he had not "been told the *inventione* [subject]" of the pictures, the same day two brothers, Camillo Ziliol and Girolamo Comin, are appointed with "the task of advising and deciding [...] on how to make and finish said pictures."

ASVe, *SGSM*, reg. 23 (Notatorio 1579–1588), c. 184; Paoletti 1929, 186

1590
August 12 – Considering that the paintings "of our Scuola [have] greatly deteriorated because of the dust," the Guardian Grande Bartolomeo Moro decides to "restore those pictures" and "make a drape" for Jacopo Tintoretto's *Miracle of the Slave*.

ASVe, *SGSM*, reg. 24 (Notatorio. 1588–1601), cc. 232r–v; Krischel 1991, 212

1591
August – * Domenico Robusti is elected *Degano mezzo anno* of the Scuola.

ASVe, *SGSM*, Atti, reg. 6 bis (Registro cariche 1440–1743), c. 17v

* The report of the voting has not been preserved. Domenico appears for the first time as *Degano mezzo anno* on April 12, 1592 (ASVe, *SGSM*, reg. 24, Notatorio 1588–1601, c. 62r)

1595
August – * Domenico Robusti is elected *Degano mezzo anno* of the Scuola.

ASVe, *SGSM*, *Atti*, reg. 6 bis (Registro cariche. 1440–1743), c. 17v

* The report of the voting has not been preserved. Domenico appears for the first time as *Degano mezzo anno* on March 11, 1596 (ASVe, *SGSM*, reg. 24, Notatorio 1588–1601, c. 118r)

1612
June 29 – Owing to the ruinous state of the chapel's altarpiece, "almost all *carolada* [worm-eaten] and tattered," the Guardian Grande Giovanni da Riva decides to entrust the commission of a new altarpiece to Domenico Tintoretto, "as he offered, and is obliged to do since the agreement of December 28, 1585" signed by his father.

ASVe, *SGSM*, reg. 25 (Notatorio 1601–12), cc. 273v–274r; Paoletti 1929, 188

1612
September 19 – In compliance with the decision taken on the date of June 29, 1612, Domenico Tintoretto is assigned the commission for the "High Altarpiece" of the chapel, to be executed according to "the Design presented by him" and with "that great diligence and refinement" promised previously by Jacopo.

ASVe, *SGSM*, reg. 26 (Notatorio 1612–23), c. 3r; Paoletti 1929, 188

1614
April 13 – Owing to the standstill in the work on the altarpiece, the Guardian Grande Girolamo Locadello decides to hold a competition in which "Signor [Domenico] Tentoretto" and "other prominent painters" will take part.

ASVe, *SGSM*, reg. 26 (Notatorio 1612–23), cc. 62r–v; S. Moschini, "Nuovi documenti sulla pala della Scuola Grande di San Marco," in *Atti dell'Istituto Veneto di scienze, lettere ed arti*, 124, (1965–66), 90

1614
June 1 – After examining "several sketches, and speaking with Signor Domenico Tentoretto and other prominent painters," Girolamo Lucadello and the Soprastanti alla Pala (Superintendents of the Altarpiece, Pietro Contarini and Fabio Lio) declare that they have reached an agreement with Jacopo Palma il Giovane for the execution of the altarpiece and its delivery by the end of "the coming month of January" for the sum of 200 *scudi*.

ASVe, *SGSM*, reg. 26 (Notatorio 1612–23), c. 66v–67r; Moschini 1965–66, 91

1614
June 27 – The Guardian Grande Girolamo Locadello receives a legal protest on the part of Perazzo Perazzi (Conservatore of the Scuola and "close relative" of Domenico Tintoretto) against the commission of the altarpiece to Jacopo Palma, considered an evident mark "of ingratitude" toward Domenico. Locadello replies to Perazzi on the same day, rebuking him for the "unwarranted and unfounded outburst," and confirming that Palma's picture "will soon be placed on the altar." Perazzi responds to this with the accusation that Locadello has caused "very grave damage to the Scuola" for having agreed to pay Palma 200 *scudi* instead of the fifty that Domenico would have requested, "working out of a sense of honor and not gain."

ASVe, *SGSM*, reg. 26 (Notatorio 1612–23), cc. 68v–70v; Moschini 1965–66, 92–95

1614
July 7 – The Guardian Grande Girolamo Lucadello puts an end to the diatribe by declaring all of Perazzo Perazzi's legal threats null and void, dismissing them as fabrications aimed at "quibbling, and fomenting undue caprices that have entered his mind."

ASVe, *SGSM*, reg. 26 (Notatorio 1612–23), c. 75v; Moschini 1965–66, 85–96

1681

April 14 – An anonymous member of the Scuola draws up the inventory of the "Quadri di Pitture nella Sala Grande" (Paintings in the Sala Grande): "Palma [il Giovane]'s altarpiece of Saint Mark on the high altar. Two pictures, one on each side of the front of said altar, one of the vision of Saint Mark in dream brought to him by the angel, the other of the blessing that the saint gave to the place where he had that vision, and where the city of Venice was to be founded. Two pictures on the left side of the aforesaid altar, one consisting of the time when the body of Saint Mark was removed from Alexandria and taken to Venetian ships. The other [with] the ships making the voyage to Venetia with the body of the aforesaid saint. Two pictures on the right side, one consisting of the storm that arose at sea during the voyage of the ships, the other the carrying in procession of that holy body from the ships to the church in Venetia in the presence of the doge and the nobility. [...] Two large pictures from the aforesaid door to the door of the main stairs, one consisting of the apparition of Saint Mark by Domenico Tintoretto son of the elder Tintoretto. The other the removal of the body of the aforesaid saint from the monuments of Alexandria with the portrait of Sir Tomaso of Ravenna former Guardian Grande of this venerable Scuola in the form of a Senator kneeling before the body lying on a rug by the elder Tintoretto. Two more pictures by the same [artist] from the door of the main stairs to the door of the Albergo, one consisting of the rain fallen from the sky at the time the Venetians carried off the body of Saint Mark, with the fear of the possessed in the presence of the aforesaid body with the spirit of the saint in the form of a cloud surrounded by angels. The other containing the miracle of Saint Mark who freed the Saracen calling on him for deliverance from the tempest at sea. [...] Between them two balconies on the front of said room where it meets the other large one. A large picture by the elder Tintoretto consisting of the miracle of the saint liberating the slave of a lord from Provence, who took a vow to come to Venetia to visit the Body of said saint against the wishes of his Master [and who] returned home was ordered by his Master to have his eyes gouged out and his bones broken with iron hammers, but all the instruments wielded to this effect broke miraculously with Saint Mark appearing in the air to free that slave to the amazement of the tyrant and the people looking on. On the side of the Rio di Santi Giovanni e Paulo meeting the stairs, between the eight openings of the balconies eight figures of sibyls painted in yellow and gold chiaroscuro."

ASVe, *SGSM*, reg. 46 (Inventario dei mobili 1681–1744), cc. 62v–63r; Paoletti 1929, 186

1690

December 13 – During the meeting of *banca* and *zonta* (auxiliary governing board) the decision is taken to restore a *penello* (processional banner) "by the hand of the celebrated painter Tentoreto the Elder."

ASVe, *SGSM*, reg. 29 (Notatorio 1684–1693), c. 224v; M. Sclosa, "Per il 'Santo Protettor nostro': il ciclo di Domenico Tintoretto alla Scuola Grande di San Marco," in *La Scuola Grande di San Marco in Venezia*, *Mirabilia Italiae* series, ed. G. Ortalli and S. Settis (Modena: Panini, 2017), 160, note 1

PAINTINGS

CAT. 1
DOMENICO TINTORETTO
(Venice, 1560–1635)
Dream of Saint Mark

c. 1587–90
Oil on canvas
314 × 388 cm
Venice, Gallerie dell'Accademia
Cat. 875

CAT. 2
DOMENICO TINTORETTO
(Venice, 1560–1635)
Saint Mark Blessing the Venetian Islands

c. 1587–90
Oil on canvas
319 × 392 cm
Venice, Gallerie dell'Accademia
In deposit at the Polo Culturale e Museale Scuola Grande di San Marco
Conservation funded by Save Venice Inc. in 2007

CAT. 3
DOMENICO TINTORETTO
(Venice, 1560–1635)
Transport of the Body of Saint Mark to the Venetian Ship

c. 1590
Oil on canvas
210 × 375 cm
Venice, Gallerie dell'Accademia
In deposit at the Polo Culturale e Museale Scuola Grande di San Marco
Conservation funded by Save Venice Inc. in 2004 (in honor of Frederick Ilchman)

CAT. 4
DOMENICO TINTORETTO
(Venice, 1560–1635)
Miracle of the Ring of Saint Mark

Late sixteenth century
Oil on canvas
400 × 370 cm
Venice, Gallerie dell'Accademia
In deposit at the Polo Culturale e Museale Scuola Grande di San Marco
Conservation funded by Save Venice Inc. in 2014

CAT. 5
DOMENICO TINTORETTO
(Venice, 1560–1635)
Arrival of the Body of Saint Mark in Venice

c. 1590–92
Oil on canvas
210 × 375 cm
Venice, Gallerie dell'Accademia
In deposit at the Polo Culturale e Museale Scuola Grande di San Marco
Conservation funded by Save Venice Inc. in 2004 (in honor of Frederick Ilchman)

CAT. 6
JACOPO NEGRETTI known as PALMA IL GIOVANE
(1548/50–1628)
Saint Mark in Glory with Saints Peter and Paul

1614–15
Oil on canvas
322 × 670 cm
Venice, Gallerie dell'Accademia
In deposit at the Polo Culturale e Museale Scuola Grande di San Marco
Conservation funded by Save Venice Inc. in 2004 (in honor of Frederick Ilchman)

CAT. 7
DOMENICO TINTORETTO
(Venice, 1560–1635)
Venice Supplicating the Virgin to Intercede with Christ to End the Plague

1631
Oil on canvas
360 × 165 cm
Venice, church of San Francesco della Vigna

II. DRAWINGS AND SKETCHES

CAT. 8
Scuola houses in the sestiere of Santa Croce

Sixteenth century
Paper, brown ink and watercolor
1040 × 420 mm
Venice, Archivio di Stato
Scuola Grande di San Marco, b. 265 (libro di disegni), allegato n. 12 (case alla Croce)

CAT. 9
DOMENICO TINTORETTO
(Venice, 1560–1635)
Origin of the Milky Way

Beginning of the seventeenth century (from original by Jacopo Tintoretto, c. 1578–80)
Pencil, bistre and watercolor on paper
252 × 356 mm
Inscription: "Do. Tintoretto"
Venice, Gallerie dell'Accademia
Inv. 121

CAT. 10
HIERONYMUS FABRICIUS
(Acquapendente, 1533–Padova, 21 May 1619)
De anatomia musculorum totius corporis

Before 1619
Oil on paper
550 × 700 mm
Venice, Biblioteca Nazionale Marciana
RARI 11. 609

CAT. 11
DOMENICO TINTORETTO
(Venice, 1560–1635)
Sketch for the *Miracle of the Ring of Saint Mark*

c. 1630
Brush in dark brown, grey, and white, on brown prepared paper
305 × 223 mm
Munich, Galerie Arnoldi-Livie

CAT. 12
GIAN AGOSTINO GRADENIGO
(Venice, 10 July 1725–Ceneda, 16 March 1774)
Medaglie di uomini illustri spettanti per lo più allo stato Viniziano con illustrazioni e disegni

Eighteenth century
Manuscript
215 × 302 × 47 mm
Venice, Biblioteca Museo Correr
Ms Cicogna 3073

CAT. 13
Perspective drawings of the Arbosani houses in Santa Croce

Second half of the eighteenth century
Paper, ink, and watercolor
550 × 380 mm
Venice, Archivio di Stato
Santa Croce di Venezia, b. 14 (unnumbered drawing)

CAT. 14
GIOVANNI GREVEMBROCH
(1731–1807)
Varie venete curiosità sacre e profane

1755
Illuminated manuscript
215 × 295 × 30 mm
Inscription: "Ospitale in Calle della Testa contrasegnato quando l'acquistò la Scuola di S. Marco"
Venice, Biblioteca Museo Correr
Ms Gradenigo Dolfin 65.1

III. ILLUMINATED MANUSCRIPTS

CAT. 15
Passio sancti Marci; Translatio Venetias sancti Marci; Apparitio seu Inventio Venetiis et miracola sancti Marci

Fourteenth century
Parchment incunable
265 × 200 mm
Venice, Biblioteca Museo Correr
Ms Correr 1498 (ms. Cl. I 416)
Conservation funded by Save Venice Inc. in 2018

CAT. 16
PAOLO VENEZIANO, attrib.
(c. 1300–c. 1365)
Illumination from the mariegola *of the Scuola Grande di San Marco*

Initiation of a Novice in the Presence of the Brethren and Saint Mark (A)
Flagellation of Christ (B)
Mid-fourteenth century
Illuminated bifolio
547 × 360 mm
Venice, Biblioteca Museo Correr
Ms Cl. IV 83
Conservation funded by Save Venice in 2018

CAT. 17
VENETIAN ILLUMINATOR
Depiction and commemorative inscription of the finding of the body of Saint Mark in the Basilica di San Marco in Venice, June 25, 1094

Mid-sixteenth century
Tempera and gold on parchment
655 × 535 mm
Venice, Museo Correr,
Gabinetto dei Disegni e delle Stampe
Inv. Cl. II, n. 24
Conservation funded by Save Venice in 2018

IV. ARCHIVAL DOCUMENTS

A. SCUOLA GRANDE DI SAN MARCO: FAITH AND HEALING

CAT. 18
Bequest for the dowries of the daughters of the Scuola members indicated in Ludovico Buora's will

1387, August 12
Paper, brown ink
225 × 290 mm
Venice, Archivio di Stato
Notarile, Testamenti, b. 557, unnumbered coupon and register of documents cc.49r-50v

CAT. 19
Agreement and convention between Leonardo Corradin and the Scuola concerning the donation of a house in calle della Testa (Santa Maria Nova) to be converted into a hospital

1491, June 17
Parchment with brown ink
413 × 640 mm
Venice, Archivio di Stato
Scuola Grande di San Marco, b. 155, fasc. A, pergamena n. 5 (Commissaria Leonardo Corradin)

CAT. 20
Nicolò Massa's admission among the doctors of the Scuola

1520
Register in parchment, leather binding, brown and colored ink
20 × 305 mm
Inscription: "Magistro Nicolò Massa a la Çerva"
Venice, Archivio di Stato
Scuola Grande di San Marco, reg. 4 (Mariegola – Elenco dei confratelli 1480-1549), cc. 98v-99r

CAT. 21
Chapter IV of the new mariegola *(statute book) for the free admission of doctors and surgeons*

c. eighteenth century (copy of original)
Sheets with paper binding, brown ink
220 × 310 mm
Venice, Archivio di Stato
Scuola Grande di San Marco, b. 216 (Parti antiche 1260–1584)

B. SCUOLA GRANDE DI SAN MARCO: TOMMASO GIANNOTTI RANGONE

CAT. 22
Admission register of noble members of the Scuola Grande di San Marco

1550–94
Paper register, parchment binding, colored ink
270 × 435 mm
Inscription (Rubrica, lettera T): "Excellente Messer Tomaxo da Ravena fixico Dottor Cavalier 1559–60 fin 73/74/75/76"
Venice, Archivio di Stato
Scuola Grande di San Marco, reg. 40, fasc. Registro nobili confratelli (I nobili, 1550-1594)

CAT. 23
Visit of Guardian Grande Tommaso Giannotti Rangone to the Scuola's hospital

1562, 3 May–1562, 14 May
Paper folder, paper binding, brown ink
230 × 330 mm
Venice, Archivio di Stato
Scuola Grande di San Marco, b. 123, fasc. A (Ospitale de poveri), cc. 30r-44r

CAT. 24
Authorization of the Guardian Grande Tommaso Giannotti Rangone to commission at his expense three canvases depicting the miracles of Saint Mark for the Sala Capitolare

1562, June 21
Paper register with leather binding, brown ink
205 × 435 × 90 mm
Venice, Archivio di Stato
Scuola Grande di San Marco, b. 22 (Notatorio 1562–1579), c. 4°

CAT. 25
Receipt given to Guardian Grande Tommaso (Giannotti Rangone) of Ravenna by Marietta born Marcantonio, wife of Andrea shoemaker of San Pietro di Castello, for the dowry of 20 ducats from Tommaso Morosini's bequest

1569, February 3
Receipt: parchment with brown ink (215 × 173 mm)
Attachments:
A. Grace: fabric; 38 × 120 mm;
Inscription: "Grazia/1568/Commissaria Morosini"

B. Wrapping : paper with brown ink
114 × 210 mm; Inscription: "La gratia de Marieta de ser Marcantonio teser in la Scuola de San Marco"
C. Marriage certificate, February 25, 1569: paper with brown ink; 155 × 218 mm
Venice, Archivio di Stato
Scuola Grande di San Marco, b. 267

CAT. 26
Will of Tommaso Giannotti Rangone

1577, 10 August –1577, 28 August
Paper folder, brown ink
225 × 320 mm
Venice, Archivio di Stato
Notarile, Testamenti, b. 421 n. 1172

CAT. 27
Record of the death of Tommaso Giannotti Rangone

1577, September 12
Paper register, brown ink
290 × 425 mm
Inscription: "12 settembre l'eccellente signor Tomaso da Ravena fo guardian grando"
Venice, Archivio di Stato
Scuola Grande di San Marco, reg. 40, fasc. Registro dei confratelli morti 1529–77, unnumbered (1577)

C. SCUOLA GRANDE DI SAN MARCO: THE CHAPEL CYCLE

CAT. 28
Agreement between Jacopo Tintoretto and the Scuola board for the execution of the painting cycle for the chapel

1585, December 28
Paper register with leather binding, brown ink
212 × 425 × 85 mm
Venice, Archivio di Stato
Scuola Grande di San Marco, reg. 23 (Notatorio 1579-1588), c. 158r

CAT. 29
Commission to Domenico Tintoretto for the altarpiece of the chapel

1612, June 29
Paper register with leather binding, brown ink
215 × 425 × 85 mm
Venice, Archivio di Stato
Scuola Grande di San Marco, reg. 25 (Notatorio 1601–12), c. 274°

CAT. 30
Commission to Jacopo Palma il Giovane for the chapel altarpiece and payment receipts

June 1, 1614 to January 28, 1615
Paper register with leather binding, brown ink
230 × 435 × 90 mm
Venice, Archivio di Stato
Scuola Grande di San Marco, reg. 26 (Notatorio 1612-1623), c. 67°

CAT. 31
Inventory of the paintings in the Sala Capitolare and the chapel

1681, April 14
Paper register with leather binding, brown ink
272 × 360 × 45 mm
Venice, Archivio di Stato
Scuola Grande di San Marco, reg. 46 (fasc. Inventario di mobili 1681–1744), cc. 62v-63r

V. ENGRAVINGS

CAT. 32
ANDREA ZUCCHI
(1679–1740)
Rescue of the Body of Saint Mark

1771 (from original by Jacopo Tintoretto, c. 1566)
Etching and burin engraving on manifold paper
645 × 469 mm
Inscription: "Temporale miracoloso sorto mentre li Alessandrini volevano impedire la Traslazione a Venezia del corpo di S. Marco / opera del Tintoretto nella sala Grande di San Marco"
Venice, Museo Correr, Gabinetto dei Disegni e delle Stampe
Inv. St.Pal.Duc. 84

VI. BOOKS

A. ANATOMY

CAT. 33
JOHANNES DE KETHAM
(fifteenth century)
In comincia el dignissimo Fasiculo de medicina in volgare el quale tracta de tute le infirmitate del corpo humano & de la anatomia de quello: & multi altri tractati composti per diuersi excelentissimi doctori con auctorita e testi prouadi

Published by Gregorio e Giovanni de' Gregori (active 1483–1516), Venice
1493 [1494]

213 × 310 mm
Venice, Biblioteca Manica Lunga, Fondazione Giorgio Cini Onlus
FOAN TES 310

CAT. 34
JACOPO BERENGARIO
(Carpi, 1466–Ferrara, 24 November 1530)
Carpi Commentaria cum amplissimis additionibus super anatomia Mundini vna cum textu eiusdem in pristinum et verum nitorem redacto

Published by Girolamo Benedetti (active 1492–1528), Bologna
1521
160 × 222 mm
Venice, Biblioteca Nazionale Marciana
199.D.175.1
Conservation funded by Save Venice Inc. in 2018

CAT. 35
JACOPO BERENGARIO
(Carpi, 1466–Ferrara, 24 November 1530)
Anatomia Carpi. Isagoge breues perlucide ac uberime, in anatomiam humani corporis, a, communi medicorum Academia, usitatam, a, Carpo in almo Bononiensi Gymnasio ordinariam chirurgiae publicae docente, ad suorum scholasticorum preces in lucem date

Published by Bernardino Vitali (active 1494–1539), Venice 1535
155 × 210 mm
Venice, Biblioteca Manica Lunga, Fondazione Giorgio Cini Onlus
FOAN TES 68

CAT. 36
ANDREAS VESALIUS
(Brussels, 31 December, 1514–Zante, 15 October 1564)
Andreae Vesalii Bruxellensis, … De humani corporis fabrica libri septem

Published by Johannes Oporinus (Basel, 25 January 1507–6 July 1568), Basel 1543
Leather binding: plates with linear frames imprinted and gilded; on the inside of the frames, and on the back plate gilded capital letters: "AND.VESALII/ANATOME" and below, separated by a gold center stamp, "THOMAS"; on the back plate, in gilded capital letters, "AND.VESALII/ EPITOME" and below, separated by a gold center stamp, "RAVENAS".
320 × 445 mm
Venice, Biblioteca Nazionale Marciana
221.D.20.1-2
Conservation funded by Save Venice Inc in 2018

CAT. 37
ANDREAS VESALIUS
(Brussels, 31 December 1514–Zante, 15 October 1564)
Andreae Vesalii Bruxellensis, scholae medicorum Patauinae professoris, suorum de humani corporis fabrica librorum Epitome

Published by Johannes Oporinus (Basel, 25 January 1507–6 July 1568), Basel 1543
350 × 505 mm
Venice, Biblioteca Nazionale Marciana
233.D.26

CAT. 38
ANDREAS VESALIUS
(Brussels, 31 Dicember 1514–Zante, 15 October 1564)
Andreae Vesalii Bruxellensis, … De humani corporis fabrica libri septem

Published by Johannes Oporinus (Basel, 25 January 1507–6 July 1568), Basel 1555
280 × 430 × 100 mm
Venice, Biblioteca di Storia della Medicina del Polo Culturale e Museale Scuola Grande di San Marco
G500 48

CAT. 39
JUAN VALVERDE DE AMUSCO
(1525–1588)
Anatomia del corpo humano composta per m. Giovan Valuerde di Hamusco, & da luy con molte figure di rame, et eruditi discorsi in luce mandata

Published by Nicolò Bevilacqua trentino (active in Venice 1554–73), Venice 1560
205 × 280 mm
Venice, Biblioteca di Storia della Medicina del Polo Culturale e Museale Scuola Grande di San Marco
G500 20
Conservation funded by Save Venice in 2018

CAT. 40
ANDREAS VESALIUS
(Brussels, 31 Dicember 1514–Zante, 15 October 1564)
Anatomes totius, aere insculpta delineatio, cui addita est Epitome innumeris mendis repurgata, quam de corporis humana conscripsit clariss. And. Vesalius: ei que accessit partium corporis tum simplicium tum compositarum breuis elucidatio, per Iacobum Greuinum Claromontanum Bellouacum, medicum Paris

Published by Andrè Wechel (active 1554–87?), Paris 1564

260 × 380 mm
Venice, Biblioteca di Storia della Medicina del Polo Culturale e Museale Scuola Grande di San Marco
G500 26

CAT. 41
IULIUS CAESAR CASSERIUS
(Piacenza, 1552–Padova, 1616)
Iulii Casseri placentini olim in Patavino gymnasio anatomiae et chirurgiae professoris celeberrimi tabulae anatomicae 78, omnes novae ante hac visae. Daniel Bucretius uratislaniensis, philos. et Med.D.20 que deorant supplevit et omnium explicationes addidit

Published by Evangelista Deuchino (active in Venice 1608–29), Venice 1627
290 × 425 mm
Venice, Biblioteca Nazionale Marciana
102.D.2
Conservation funded by Save Venice in 2018

B. SURGERY

CAT. 42
JOHANNES DE KETHAM
(fifteenth century)
Fasciculus medicinae. Similitudo complexionum & elementorum

Published by Gregorio de Gregori (active 1480–1528), Venice 1491
280 × 405 mm
Venice, Biblioteca Manica Lunga, Fondazione Giorgio Cini Onlus
FOAN TES 309

CAT. 43
JEAN TAGAULT
(c. 1486–1546)
Ioannis Tagaultii ... De chirurgica institutione libri quinque. His accessit sextus liber de materia chirurgica, authore Iacobo Hollerio ... unà cum indice copiosissiomo

Published by Vincenzo Valgrisi (active in Venice 1539–73), Venice 1549
120 × 170 × 40 mm
Venice, Biblioteca di Storia della Medicina del Polo Culturale e Museale Scuola Grande di San Marco
P500 56
Conservation funded by Save Venice in 2018

CAT. 44
CLAUDIUS GALENUS
(Pergamon, 129–Rome or Pergamon 201)
[8]: *Galeni Septima classis. Curandi methodum tum diffuse tum breuiter descriptam, uictus rationem in morbis acutis, singularum morborum facile paranda remedia, priuatam quorundam morborum curationem, chirurgiae constitutionem, fracturarum ac luxationum sanationem, fasciarum denique & laqueorum & machinamentorum tractatum continet. ... Tò therapeutikón*

Published by heirs of Lucantonio Giunta (active in Venice 1535–69), Venice 1550
255 × 360 × 70 mm
Venice, Biblioteca di Storia della Medicina del Polo Culturale e Museale Scuola Grande di San Marco
G500 5/3

CAT. 45
CLAUDIUS GALENUS
(Pergamon, 129–Rome or Pergamon, 201)
Galeni Omnia, quae extant singulari studio, summaq. diligentia Io. Baptistae Rasarii emendata, nouo ordine cuius etiam attulimus rationem, disposita, librorum nuper inuentorum accessione aucta, & magna ex parte in Latinam linguam conuersa.

Published by Vincenzo Valgrisi (active Venice 1539–73), Venice 1562–63
328 × 365 mm
Venice, Biblioteca Nazionale Marciana
126.D.5
Conservation funded by Save Venice in 2018

CAT. 46
JEAN TAGAULT
(c. 1486–1546)
Ioan. Tagaultii ... De chirurgica institutione libri quinque. His accessit sextus liber de materia chirurgica, authore Iacobo Hollerio ...

Published by Guillame Rouillé (active 1545–89), Lione 1567
115 × 170 × 30 mm
Venice, Biblioteca di Storia della Medicina del Polo Culturale e Museale Scuola Grande di San Marco
P500 59

CAT. 47
GIOVANNI ANDREA DALLA CROCE
(Venice, 1515?–1575)
Chirurgiae Ioannis Andreae a Cruce, Veneti medici libri septem, quamplurimis instrumentorum imaginibus arti chirurgicae opportunis suis locis exornati, theoricam, practicam, ac uerissimam experientiam

continentes. In quibus ea omnia, quae optimo chirurgo in curandis vulneribus conuenire videntur, ordine quodam amplissimo concerni possunt nunc primum in lucem editi

Published by Giordano Ziletti
(active 1549–1583), Venice 1573
220 × 300 × 25 mm
Bologna, Donazione Putti, Istituto Ortopedico Rizzoli
IF 22

CAT. 48
GIOVANNI DA VIGO
(Rapallo, 1450–Rome, 1525)
La pratica vniuersale in cirugia di m. Giouanni di Vico genouese. Di nuouo ristampata, & corretta. Appresso vi è vn bellissimo compendio, che tratta dell'istessa materia, composto per m. Mariano Santo barolitano. Con due trattati di m. Gio. Andrea dalla Croce, l'vno in materia delle ferite, l'altro del cauar l'armi, e le saette fuori della carne. Con alcuni strumenti in disegno. Et di nuouo aggiuntiui molti capitoli estratti dalle opere dell'eccellentissimo dottor, & caualier, il sig. Leonardo Fiorauanti bolognese, i quali sono molto necessarij alla medicina, & cirugia per bene operare ...

Published by Giovanni Maria Bonelli il Giovane (active in Venice from 1575), Venice 1576
170 × 215 × 55 mm
Venice, Biblioteca di Storia della Medicina del Polo Culturale e Museale Scuola Grande di San Marco
M500 28

CAT. 49
GIOVANNI ANDREA DALLA CROCE
(Venice, 1515–1575)
Cirugia vniuersale e perfetta di tutte le parti pertinenti all'ottimo chirurgo. Di Gio. Andrea Dalla Croce medico vinitiano. Nellaquale si contiene la theorica, & prattica di ciò che può essere nella cirugia necessario: come più ampiamente nel sommario si dichiara. Di nuouo con li dissegni di tutti gl'istromenti antichi & moderni in tal'arte necessarij, posta in luce. Con la tauola de' capitoli di ciascun libro

Published by Giordano Ziletti
(active 1549–83), Venice
1583
225 × 310 × 70 mm
Bologna, Donazione Putti, Istituto Ortopedico Rizzoli
IF 18

CAT. 50
AMBROISE PARÉ
(Bourg–Hersent, Laval, 1510–Paris, 20 December 1590)
Opera chirurgica Ambrosij Paraei, Galliarum regis primarij, et Parisiensis chirurgi. Quibus continentur, non solum perfectissima curandi ratio tumores praeter naturam, vulnera, vlcera, luxationes, & fracturas: ... A docto viro, plerisque locis recognita: & latinitate donata. Iacobi Guillemeau, ... labore & diligentia. Omnia nunc demum magno studio elimata: et nouis iconibus elegantissimis illustrata

Published by Johann Feyerabend
(active 1573–99) and Peter Fischer (?-1595), Frankfurt 1594
240 × 355 × 75 mm
Venice, Biblioteca di Storia della Medicina del Polo Culturale e Museale Scuola Grande di San Marco
G500 18

CAT. 51
JEAN TAGAULT
(c. 1486–1546)
Institutione di cirugia di Giovanni Tagaultio medico illustre, distinta in libri cinque. Aggiuntoui il sesto libro della materia di cirugia, di Giacomo Hollerio ... Con due tauole l'una de' capitoli; l'altra, delle cose degne di memoria

Published by Nicolò Moretti
(active 1583–1608), Venice
1596
115 × 150 × 55 mm
Venice, Biblioteca di Storia della Medicina del Polo Culturale e Museale Scuola Grande di San Marco
P500 79

C. PLAGUE

CAT. 52
JOHANNES DE KETHAM
(fifteenth century)
Incipit fasciculus medicine compositus per excellentissimum artium ac medicine doctorem dominum Joannem de Ketam alamanum: tractans de anothomia ... cui annectuntur multi alij tractatus per diuersos excellentissimos doctores compositi. Necnon anothomia Mundini...

Published by Gregorio de Gregori
(active 1480–1528), Venice 1513
215 × 308 mm
Venice, Biblioteca Manica Lunga, Fondazione Giorgio Cini Onlus
FOAN TES 311

CAT. 53
NICCOLÒ MASSA
(Venice, 14 March 1489–27 August 1569)
Nicolai Massa ... Liber de febre pestilentiali, ac de pestichiis, morbillis, variolis, & apostematibus pestilentialibus, ac eorundem omnium curatione, necnon de modo quo corporà peste praeseruari debeant. ... Cum indice rerum notabilium ...

Published by Andrea Arrivabene
(active in Venice 1534–70), Venice 1556
160 × 210 mm
Venice, Biblioteca di Storia della Medicina del Polo Culturale e Museale Scuola Grande di San Marco
M500 15

CAT. 54
PIETRO ANDREA MATTIOLI
(Siena, 12 March 1501–Trent, 1578)
Petri Andreae Matthioli Senensis medici, Commentarii in sex libros Pedacii Dioscoridis Anazarbei de medica materia, iam denuo ab ipso autore recogniti, et locis plus mille aucti. Adiectis magnis, ac nouis plantarum, ac animalium iconibus, supra priores editiones longè pluribus, ad uiuum delineatis.\Georgius Liberalis & Volfangus Meierpeck! Accesserunt quoque ad margines Graeci contextus quàm plurimi, ex antiquissimis codicibus desumpti, qui Dioscoridis ipsius deprauatam lectionem restituunt. Cum locupletissimis indicibus, tum ad rem herbariam, tum medicamentariam pertinentibus

Published by Vincenzo Valgrisi
(active in Venice 1539–73), Venice 1565
275 × 380 × 110 mm
Venice, Biblioteca di Storia della Medicina del Polo Culturale e Museale Scuola Grande di San Marco
G500 43

CAT. 55
TOMMASO GIANNOTTI RANGONE
(Ravenna, August 1493–Venice, 10 September 1577)
Serenissimo principi d.d. Sebastiano Venerio inclyto Venetorum, et, c. [*sic*] *duci sapientissimo. Thomas philologus Rangonus Rauennas ... De vita principis, et Venetorum commoda semper: consilium*

Published *all'insegna della Regina*
(active in Venice 1557–99), Venice 1577
150 × 160 mm
Venice, Biblioteca di Storia della Medicina del Polo Culturale e Museale Scuola Grande di San Marco
P500 46
Conservation funded by Save Venice in 2018

D. FAITH AND DEVOTION

CAT. 56
Questa operetta tracta dellarte del ben morire cioe in gratia di Dio

Published by Giovan Battista Sessa
(active in Venice 1489–1509), Venice 1503
145 × 197 mm
Venice, Biblioteca Manica Lunga, Fondazione Giorgio Cini Onlus
FOAN TES 748

CAT. 57
Libro da compagnia o vero di fraternita di battuti nouamente stampato: & diligentemente correcto con molte aditione a laude de dio & de la gloriosa virgine maria; & de li deuoti christiani. Et historiato

Published by Nicolò Zoppino di Aristotile de' Rossi and Vincenzo di Paolo
(active in Venice 1513–24), Venice
1518, 22 September
160 × 215 mm
Venice, Biblioteca Manica Lunga, Fondazione Giorgio Cini Onlus
FOAN TES 669

CAT. 58
GIROLAMO SAVONAROLA
(21 September 1452–23 May 1498)
Predica del arte del bene morire

Published by Bartolomeo de' Libri
(active 1482–c. 1520) and Giovanni Stefano di Carlo (active 1505?–1521), Florence
1515–30
140 × 205 mm
Venice, Biblioteca Manica Lunga, Fondazione Giorgio Cini Onlus
FOAN TES 829

E. ART

CAT. 59
ODOARDO FIALETTI
(Bologna, 18 July 1573–Venice, 1636/38)
Il uero modo et ordine. Per dissegnar tutte le parti. Et membra del corpo humano. Di Odoardo Fialetti pittor

Published by Justus Sadeler (1572?–1620?), Venice
1608
245 × 180 mm
Venice, Biblioteca Nazionale Marciana
41.D.199
Conservation funded by Save Venice in 2018

CAT. 60
GIACOMO FRANCO
(1550–Venice, 28 June 1620)
Regole per imparar a disegnar i corpi humani diuise in doi libri delineati dal famoso pittor Giacomo Palma

First book: published by Marco Sadeler (1616–60), Venice 1636
Second book: published by Stefano Scolari (active in Venice 1644–87), Venice 1659
Burin engraving and etching
280 × 375 mm
Venice, Biblioteca Nazionale Marciana
40.D.19
Conservation funded by Save Venice in 2018

CAT. 61
GASPARO COLOMBINA
(Padua, early 1580s–Udine, 1651)
Discorso sopra il modo di disegnare. dipingere, & spiegare secondo l'una, & l'altr'arte gli affetti principali

Published by Giovanni Temini (active 1589–?), Padua
c. 1650
220 × 305 mm
Venice, Biblioteca Nazionale Marciana
31.D.4
Conservation funded by Save Venice in 2018

F. MUSIC

CAT. 62
CLAUDIO MONTEVERDI
(Cremona, 9 May 1567–Venice 29 November 1643)
Selva Morale e Spirituale di Claudio Monteverde Maestro di Capella della Serenissima Republica Di Venetia Dedicata alla Sacra Cesarea Maesta dell'Imperatrice Eleonora Gonzaga Con Licenza de Superiori & Priuilegio ... in 4°. Soprano primo, Soprano secondo, Alto primo, Alto e Basso secondo, Tenore primo, Tenore secondo, Basso primo, (il Basso secondo è compreso nella parte dell'Alto surriferita), Violino primo, Violino secondo, e Basso continuo. In tutto dieci grossi libercoli.

Published by Bartolomeo Magni (Ravenna, second half of the sixteenth century–?), Venice
1640
Height 22.5 cm, width 16,8 cm
Museo Internazionale e Biblioteca della Musica di Bologna
BB.13 (facsimile)

VII. WOODCUT BLOCKS

CAT. 63
Scene of an anatomical manipulation

Wooden block
Used to print *Claudius Galenus, Galeni Omnia, quae extant singulari studio, summaq. diligentia Io. Baptistae Rasarii emendata, nouo ordine cuius etiam attulimus rationem, disposita, librorum nuper inuentorum accessione aucta, & magna ex parte in Latinam linguam conuersa*, Vincenzo Valgrisi, Venice 1562
Tomo V, *In Hippocratem de fracturis*, p. 249r
Mid-sixteenth century
12 × 7,2 cm
Venice, Museo Correr
Inv. Cl. XXXIII, s.n. 222

CAT. 64
Scene of an anatomical manipulation

Wooden block
Used to print *Claudius Galenus, Galeni Omnia, quae extant singulari studio, summaq. diligentia Io. Baptistae Rasarii emendata, nouo ordine cuius etiam attulimus rationem, disposita, librorum nuper inuentorum accessione aucta, & magna ex parte in Latinam linguam conuersa*, Vincenzo Valgrisi, Venice 1562
Tomo V, *In Hippocratem de fracturis*, p. 263v
Mid-sixteenth century
12 × 7,2 cm
Venice, Museo Correr
Inv. Cl. XXXIII, s.n. 225

CAT. 65
Scene of an anatomical manipulation

Wooden block
Used to print *Claudius Galenus, Galeni Omnia, quae extant singulari studio, summaq. diligentia Io. Baptistae Rasarii emendata, nouo ordine cuius etiam attulimus rationem, disposita, librorum nuper inuentorum accessione aucta, & magna ex parte in Latinam linguam conuersa*, Vincenzo Valgrisi, Venice 1562
Tomo V, *In Hippocratem de articulis*, p. 282r
Mid-sixteenth century
11,7 × 6 cm
Venice, Museo Correr
Inv. Cl. XXXIII, s.n. 221

CAT. 66
Scene of an anatomical manipulation

Wooden block
Used to print *Claudius Galenus, Galeni Omnia, quae extant singulari studio, summaq. diligentia Io. Baptistae Rasarii emendata, nouo ordine cuius etiam attulimus rationem, disposita, librorum nuper inuentorum accessione aucta, & magna ex parte in Latinam linguam conuersa*, Vincenzo Valgrisi, Venice 1562
Tomo V, *In Hippocratem de articulis*, p. 297v
Mid-sixteenth century
12 × 6 cm
Venice, Museo Correr
Inv. Cl. XXXIII, s.n. 224

CAT. 67
Scene of an anatomical manipulation

Wooden block
Used to print *Claudius Galenus, Galeni Omnia, quae extant singulari studio, summaq. diligentia Io. Baptistae Rasarii emendata, nouo ordine cuius etiam attulimus rationem, disposita, librorum nuper inuentorum accessione aucta, & magna ex parte in Latinam linguam conuersa*, Vincenzo Valgrisi, Venice 1562
Tomo V, *In Hippocratem de fracturis*, p. 248r
Mid-sixteenth century
12,3 × 7,2 cm
Venice, Museo Correr
Inv. Cl. XXXIII, s.n. 226

VIII. MEDALS

CAT. 68
Badge of the Scuola Grande di San Marco

Sixteenth century
Cast bronze
g 2,05, Ø mm 23
Venice, Museo Correr,
Gabinetto di Numismatica
Inv. Tessere 158

CAT. 69
Badge of the Scuola Grande di San Marco

Sixteenth century
Cast bronze
Venice, Museo Correr,
Gabinetto di Numismatica
Inv. Tessere 157

CAT. 70
Badge of the Scuola Grande di San Marco

Sixteenth century
Cast bronze
Venice, Museo Correr,
Gabinetto di Numismatica
Inv. Tessere 157

CAT. 71
MATTEO PAGANO, attrib.
(known from 1543)
Magnum medal depicting the *Origin of the Milky Way* (verso)

c. 1560
Cast bronze
g 24, 81, Ø mm 40, h 12 mm
Inscription: "A.IOVE.ET.SORORE. GENITA."
Venice, Museo Correr,
Gabinetto di Numismatica
Cl. XXIX n. 1498

CAT. 72
MATTEO PAGANO, attrib.
(documented from 1543)
Magnum medal with a *Portrait of Tommaso Giannotti Rangone* (recto)

1562
Bronze
g 23, 21, Ø mm 40, h 12 mm
Inscription: "D/THOM[AS]. PHILOL[OGUS].RAVEN[NAS]. PHYS[ICVS].EQ[VES] GVARD[IANVS].D[IVI].MAR[CI]. MAG[ISTE]"; to the left of the bust: "1562"
Venice, Museo Correr,
Gabinetto di Numismatica
Cl. XXIX n. 245

IX. SURGICAL INSTRUMENTS

CAT. 73
Cranium drill and bits

Sixteenth century
Wood and metal
Drill: 11 × 27 cm
Bits: 2 × 9 cm
Bologna, Donazione Putti,
Istituto Ortopedico Rizzoli

CAT. 74
Bone scraper

Sixteenth century
Wood and metal
4,5 × 18 cm
Bologna, Donazione Putti,
Istituto Ortopedico Rizzoli

CAT. 75
Bone saw

Sixteenth century
Wood and metal
8 × 46 cm
Bologna, Donazione Putti,
Istituto Ortopedico Rizzoli

CAT. 76
Perforator

Sixteenth century
Wood and metal
3,5 × 13,5 cm
Bologna, Donazione Putti,
Istituto Ortopedico Rizzoli

Photo Credits
2018 © Archivio Fotografico - Fondazione Musei Civici di Venezia: cat. 15 p. 25, cat. 16A-B p. 33, cat. 69 p. 34, cat. 70 p. 34, cat. 14 p. 37, cat. 71 p. 46, cat. 72 p. 46, cat. 63 p. 113.
Archivio Scuola Grande di San Rocco / © Cameraphoto Arte®, Venice: fig. 10 p. 58, fig. 10 p. 61.
© Arnoldi-Livie, München: cat. 11 p. 89.
Biblioteca Nazionale Marciana, Venice, su concessione del Ministero dei beni e delle attività culturali e del turismo. Divieto di riproduzione: cat. 36 p. 53, cat. 36 pp. 54–55, fig. 11 p. 62, cat. 36 p. 74, cat. 36 p. 78, cat. 10 p. 79, cat 59 p. 81, cat. 59 p. 84, cat. 59 p. 86, cat. 45 p. 112, cat. 59 pp. 116–7.
© Cameraphoto Arte®, Venice: fig. 1 p. 16, fig. 2 p. 18, cat. 3 p. 21, cat. 5 p. 21, cat. 6 p. 22, cat. 2 p. 23, cat. 4 p. 24.
Diocesi Patriarcato di Venezia, Ufficio Beni Culturali: cat. 7 p. 68, cat. 7 p. 71.
Fondazione Giorgio Cini Onlus, Venice: cat. 57 p. 30, cat. 33 p. 78, cat. 52 p. 104, cat. 42 p. 107, cat. 35 p. 108.
Gabinetto Fotografico delle Gallerie degli Uffizi, Florence: fig. 14 p. 88.
© Istituto Ortopedico Rizzoli, Bologna, Donazione Putti: cat. 49 p. 27, cat. 73 p. 27, cat. 49 p. 97, cat. 73 p. 97, cat. 49 p. 97, cat. 49 p. 99.
© Matteo De Fina, Venice: fig. 8 p. 52, cat. 57 p. 30, cat. 7 p. 68, cat. 7 p. 71, cat. 38 p. 76, cat. 33 p. 78, cat. 39 p. 79, fig. 18 p. 94, cat. 44 p. 96, cat. 50 p. 100, cat. 52 p. 104, cat. 42 p. 107, cat. 35 p. 108, cat. 38 p. 108, cat. 51 p. 111.
Michelle Laughran fig. 9 p. 60.
Museo Nazionale Gallerie dell'Accademia di Venezia, © Archivio fotografico G.A.VE, su concessione del Ministero dei beni e delle attività culturali e del turismo: fig. 4 p. 19, cat. 1 p. 20, cat. 9 p. 47, fig. 6 p. 42, fig. 6 p. 48, fig. 7 p. 50.
Pinacoteca di Brera, Milan © 2018. Foto Scala, Florence - su concessione Ministero dei beni e delle attività culturali e del turismo fig. 3 p. 14, fig. 3 p. 18.
Polo Culturale e Museale Scuola Grande di San Marco, Venice: cat. 44 pp. 12–13, fig. 1 p. 16, fig. 2 p. 18, cat. 3 p. 21, cat. 5 p. 21, cat. 6 p. 22, cat. 2 p. 23, cat. 4 p. 24, cat. 38 p. 76, cat. 39 p. 79, fig. 18 p. 94, cat. 44 p. 96, cat. 50 p. 100, cat. 38 p. 108, cat. 51 p. 111.
© 2017. Princeton University Art Museum / Art Resource NY/Scala, Florence: fig. 13 p. 71.
© RMN-Grand Palais (Museé du Louvre) / Michel Urtado: fig. 16 p. 90.
Shylock e-solutions, Venice: cat. 36 p. 53, cat. 36 pp. 54–55, cat. 36 p. 74, cat. 36 p. 78, cat. 45 p. 112.
© The Pierpont Morgan Library, New York: fig. 15 pp. 88–89.
© Victoria and Albert Museum, London: fig. 5 p. 23.
Wellcome Library, London: (CC BY 4.0: https://creativecommons.org/licenses/by/4.0/): fig. 12 p. 65.

Repro
Opero s.r.l., Verona

Printing
Grafiche Veneziane s.r.l., Venezia
for Marsilio Editori® s.p.a. in Venezia